BAD GRANDMA AND OTHER CHAPTERS IN A LIFE LIVED OUT LOUD

Elaine Soloway

ISBN: 1542480019
ISBN 13: 9781542480017

Photo by Ron Gould Studios

Also by Elaine Soloway

The Division Street Princess

She's Not The Type

Green Nails and Other Acts of Rebellion: Life After Loss

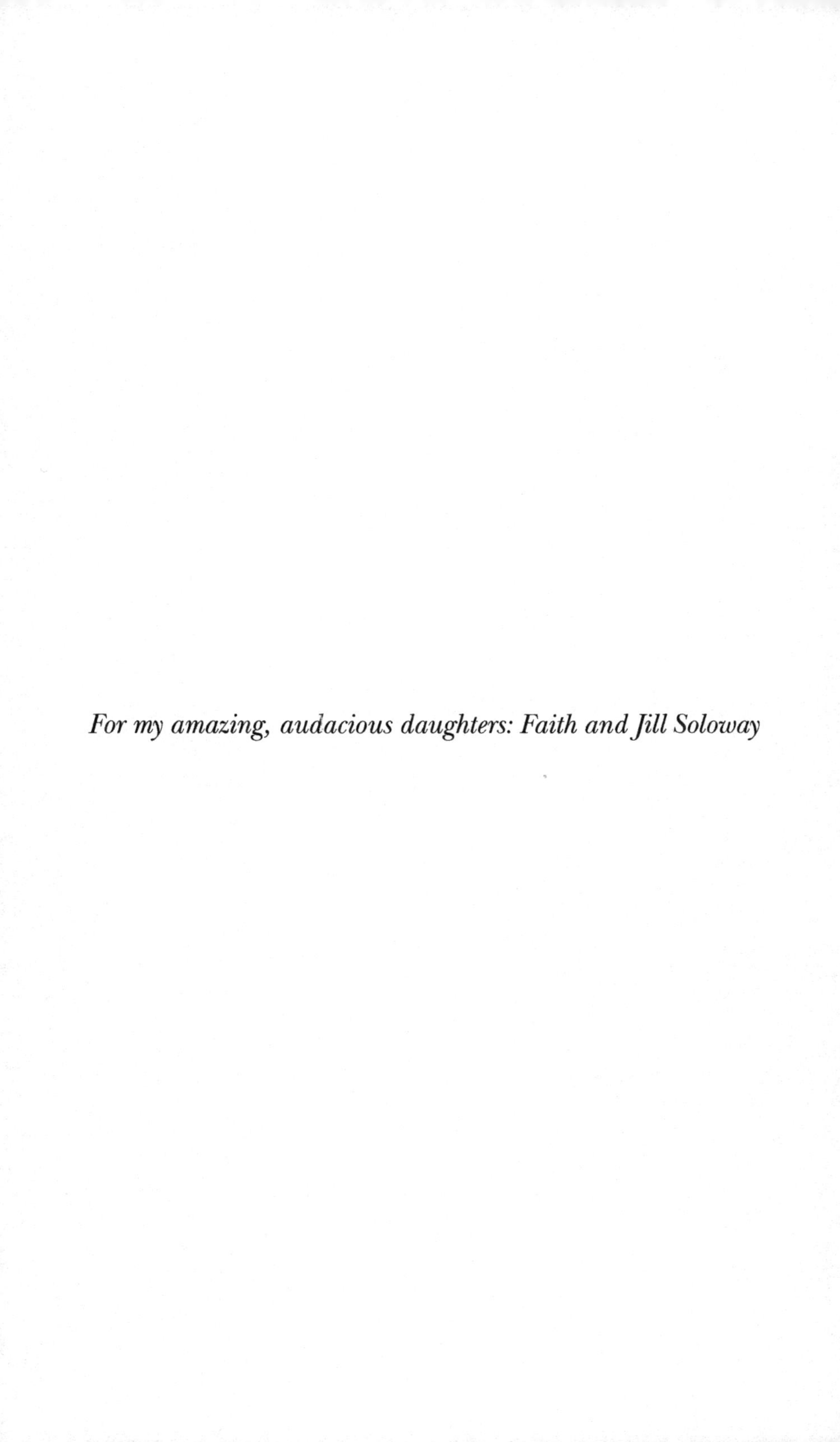

For my amazing, audacious daughters: Faith and Jill Soloway

TABLE OF CONTENTS

DRIVING MS. ELAINE

I watched as car after car slipped through the half moon driveway of my apartment building. I was on the lookout for a silver Passat station wagon that was being driven by a young woman assigned to pick me up for a holiday event.

The driver and the other women in the car were unknown to me, but we had a mutual friend, and it was this kind soul who had given the female crew my name, address, and instructions.

When the Passat arrived, I spun through the lobby's revolving door, and as I landed on the other side, realized I had also been transformed. I had now become a version of *The Elderly Aunt Who Needs A Ride.*

"Hi, thanks so much for picking me up," I said to the driver.

"My pleasure," she said.

As we rode, I was desperate to erase the unpleasant label I had given myself. I wouldn't sit dumbly as if I were being chauffeured, but instead be friendly and inquisitive. "So, what do you do?" I posed to the car's occupants, and listened as each drew a picture of their lives.

But as they responded, I couldn't focus because a figure from my past came knocking on the door of my brain.

"I'm disappointed in you, Princess. I never thought you'd give up driving; never thought I've find you in the back seat." It was my father, Irv, who taught me how to drive when I was a teen. Dad died in 1958, and although many decades have passed since then, he has visited me often to praise or needle.

It was tricky trying to take in the women's responses with my dad nagging in the background, but I was eager to defend myself. "I didn't give up driving," I said to him, "I just no longer own a car. It was too expensive, and..."

"Do you remember my Buick?" Dad interrupted. "I think we had to use three pillows to get you up over the steering wheel."

In my imagination, I saw him take a drag of his Camel cigarette. I was about to reach over to the window to let the smoke out, but stopped when I realized I'd be accommodating an illusion.

"Of course I remember your car," I said, certain to reply silently so that the other riders wouldn't think I was indeed a doddering old aunt. "And you know what I remember most about the drives," I said, "your arms."

"You mean because they were so powerful from the swimming I did at the Y?" Dad said. I could see him preening, growing taller than his 5'4" stature and even slimmer than his Santa-like shape.

"No, Dad," I said, "I remember your arms because your left was tanned from the tip of your fingers to your elbow, while the upper part was chalky white. You always had that arm out the window so you could flick ashes."

"Not when I was teaching you," Dad said, reminding me of his crucial tutoring role.

"No, when you were teaching me, you were using the overflowing ashtray and pounding an imaginary brake at each light."

Dad laughed. I saw his brown eyes brighten, the thin mustache that almost looked penciled in, and a smile that revealed teeth I saw nightly floating in a drinking glass. The image of him was so vivid I could almost smell the cigarette's smoke.

Our real life driver had reached our destination and was about to park. "Let's watch, Dad," I said, "let's see if she can do this in one shot."

The driver positioned her Passat alongside of the car in front of the empty space. Dad and I stared, but he couldn't resist coaching: "As you back up, turn the steering wheel to the right. Fix your eyes on the right headlight of the car parked behind. Aim for your target, and then reverse the direction of the steering wheel."

This time, it was my turn to laugh. "That's the way you taught me to how to parallel park. You know I passed it on to your granddaughters and then to your great grandson."

"We're here," the women chorused. As the three of them exited the car and were walking to the restaurant's entrance, I lagged behind. “Time to go, Dad,” I said. “But, you can see one major advantage of giving up driving: I don’t have to concentrate on the road, so I can let my mind wander.”

“You mean we can continue on the ride home?” Dad said.

“Count on it.”

ABSTINENCE

Gerry tosses a green beach ball -- the color of a lime Popsicle -- to Anna. Although she is seated in a wheelchair, Anna is able to catch the ball, which is slowly deflating and becoming cushy, and send it back to the physical therapist.

I have joined the half-circle of six hospital patients who are participating in this mild exercise class. My friend, Louise, who has a broken right arm, is seated next to me.

I am able-bodied, but am allowed to accompany my longtime friend because she threatened to skip the session to have more time with me.

After class, when Louise choses a chair for her lunchtime, I perch on her hospital bed and attempt to cheer her. *The old gray mare, she ain't what she used to be,* Louise sings as I remove the heavy cover from her vegetarian meal. As I cut the grain burger into fourths to make it easier for her to do a one-armed grab, I remind her, *you'll recover and go home soon.* I am trying to dissuade her from a track that typically veers from the ditty to depression.

As our conversation continues, several thoughts hit me: *I am good at this* and surprisingly, *I enjoy caregiving.*

Then, a scary one bubbles up: Could this sense of enjoyment propel me towards a new male in need of rehabilitation rather than an able-bodied one?

What if I haven't shucked enough of the comfort and care I had bestowed on my late husband, and have leftover succor that seeks a target?

That question frightened me so much, that on the spot, I made a resolution: To avoid falling for a failing fellow, I would abstain from getting involved with any male. I would give up the idea of dating; for surely, with my proclivity for caring, I couldn't be trusted.

Just then, I felt a soft tap on my shoulder. The touch was so tender I knew it wasn't real or earthbound, but instead, coming from a deceased loved one. It couldn't be Tommy because I knew he avoids topics where other males are involved. And, I had recently gabbed with both my mother and father. So, who was it that wanted a word in on my latest vow?

"Sweetheart," came the familiar voice.

"Rita?" I said. "It's great to hear from you. This is the first time you've come down to chat since you died 14 years ago. I'm thrilled to have your presence, but why now?"

"Just because you haven't heard from me doesn't mean we're not in each other's thoughts. I notice you dream about me quite a bit. And you wrote about me in your roman a clef, 'She's Not The Type,' right?"

"You read that?" I said.

"It's an eBook, so I read it on iCloud. Loved your description of me: *Rita had dark hair cut in a pageboy, eyes almost too big for her small face, earrings that overwhelmed her tiny lobes, and she wore a suit with shoulder pads that widened her slim figure.*"

"You memorized it!"

"Who wouldn't?" she said. "Listen, the reason for my visit is I heard you declare you were abstaining from men. Is that true, or did the words get garbled when they travelled between earth and heaven?"

Of course, it would be gorgeous, male-attracting Rita concerned about my total avoidance of the opposite sex. My dear friend was never without a good-looking, fun-loving guy at her side.

"I think it's for my own good," I said. "I realize I like caregiving. Sure, there were times with Tommy when fear and weariness took over, but generally, I got pleasure from it. I'm afraid I'll find myself back in a situation that can only end badly. Why not avoid it altogether and be solo for the rest of my life?"

"What about excitement, passion? Surely there's a spark left?"

"Rita, dearest," I said. "Up there, you're still a comely 67 or maybe younger. Down here, I'm a shrinking 75. And, I'm not only talking about height, but also libido."

"Stop, shush," she said. "That attitude is verboten up here."

"You mean..."

"Of course, we're still horny in heaven. In fact, I've got a date tonight, so I have to say so long."

"Anyone I know?"

"Think matinee idol." she said.

"Cary Grant? Marlon Brando?"

I heard Rita's adorable laugh; and then silence; she was gone, likely primping for her date.

Instead of considering Rita's view, I chose the couch and the remote. Here, my boyfriend Netflix and I cuddled, where the only caregiving required is a switch from Cable to HDMI2.

A STRONG SOMEBODY

My bitsy lime green kitchen table -- which is not really in the kitchen, but is adjacent to the living room window -- has been cleared of placemats and flowerpots. Atop the surface is a file marked "Taxes 2013" and a workbook that requires my input before returning it to my accountant.

Although the view from the empty chair at the table is quite lovely with the sun rising over the river, the message I'm receiving is: *get over here, sit down, and get to work.* I rebut this with: *I wish I had a strong somebody to take over and tackle the taxes.*

It's not only the looming paperwork that has me down and desperate, but also several recent episodes that have my strong facade fracturing and seeking a rescuer.

Consider: I returned home from a four-day trip to Los Angeles and was greeted by a warning from my fund manager that my email account had been hacked. "Did you really want to wire transfer $$, $$$ to Hong Kong?" he asked.

Instead of a soft homecoming where I could ease into my benign routine, I plunged into changing passwords, adding security locks to open cyber doors, alerting my bank, and checking with the Chicago police. All this activity occurred while my suitcase glared unpacked and the washing machine yawned empty of the weekend's laundry.

"It's great that you know how to do all of that computer stuff," said a friend. While she surely wanted to buck me up for slippery roads still ahead, all I could think of was: *I wish I had a strong somebody to protect me.*

Perhaps the positive image I've created of a self-sufficient former caregiver, current widow dazzles some. But at times, I feel fraudulent, like the wizard behind the curtain. If one of my fans were to draw back the drapery, instead of a towering landing-on-her-feet damsel, they'd find a tiny, elderly, frightened female.

Oh, do I sound like I'm feeling sorry for myself? Hey, I'm allowed. Take the recent airline travel as example. Fortunately, American Airlines has seen through my disguise and granted me Expedited Boarding. This allows me to more speedily enter the gates and keep my laptop or cosmetic bag stowed. (Boots still have to go.) But, where was a strong somebody to hoist my luggage onto the conveyor belt? And, after a flight attendant turned me down with, *Bad back; you'll have to find somebody's husband,* I did just that.

"Could you?" I said to the first tall male in the aisle. His wife gave me a look, which I interpreted as *Find your own strong somebody*, but the guy ignored her and fulfilled my request.

Perhaps I got spoiled in Los Angeles where both of my daughters stepped in to act as strong somebodies when my emotional and physical health needed babying. The eldest took me for a walk to allow me to unplug some bruised feelings. And the youngest brewed tea to sooth my cold and packed a lunch for my next-day flight. While I know the situation should be reversed, and I should be the one pampering my kids, it was delicious to be on the other end of the caregiving model.

And I suppose if I surveyed my current life, rather than a strong somebody supervising my apartment needs, I've got an entire maintenance crew and concierge staff tending to me.

Already, I feel myself hoisted -- something like the suitcase in the overhead that can shift in flight -- out of self -pity, and moving towards the light. In my imagination, I open a door marked Blessings and find a room crowded with friends and relatives. Basking in the glow of recovery, I see each one wears a hat. (Could be a crown if you prefer historical or biblical references.) While the headpieces are varied, the messages atop are alike: Strong Somebody is the imprint.

In the film clip I'm creating, there's a soundtrack with triumphant music as I realize I am not absent a rescuer, but instead are surrounded with many. "You are the strongest of us all," I hear one friend shout. I beam and accept the empty chair (Let's get the prop from my kitchen table.), which they use to hoist me above the crowd.

I look around as I'm carried and off to the side, I see a closed curtain. From my height, I yell, "Draw it open!"

You guessed it: the tiny, elderly, frightened female has vanished, and in her place is my new mirror image. The Strongest Somebody of them all.

A NEW LEASE

I've raised the horizontal blinds that cover the floor-to-ceiling windows of my convertible studio apartment. The Chicago River is frozen over, cars on the expressway are slogging in both directions, and the sun is sneaking above the high-rise and loft buildings that complete my view to the north.

A new lease waiting to be approved is on my small Lime Ricky green table. As of April 15, I will have lived here for one year. I settle on a pillow that softens the seat of a wooden chair and start reviewing before I sign on the dotted line.

The view distracts me, so I drop my pen and allow myself to muse over the decision I made just two months after my husband died November 2, 2012. Elbowing past advice to make no major moves for at least a year, I put our house on the market. And five months later I landed here, in this new apartment and life. Now, as the lease renewal approaches, I decide it's time to review the pros and cons, and changes, which have occurred since that swift transition.

First the pros:
I love my living space. While the views are new, the furnishings are warmly familiar. A dozen paintings that burst our house's walls with color and interest are now hanging in my 612-foot-cocoon.

My Kingsbury Plaza maintenance men leveled, nailed, and attached all; one of many tasks they have undertaken with sweet eagerness.

I am typing this essay on a gaunt MacBook Air, which I exchanged for a muscular desktop that would've overwhelmed my Sapphire blue worktable and pint-sized apartment. Instead of the home office I once had, I now work in a snug corner with a built-in bookshelf that holds the few volumes, photographs, mementoes, and supplies I brought with.

I am managing without owning a car. A major change between my former life and current -- other than I'm absent my husband -- is that I no longer own a car. Finances were the primary reason, but also, I can walk to grocery and department stores, am a few blocks from three CTA lines, and can hail taxicabs or use an App for shared rides.

I have boosted my physical and spiritual health. The East Bank Club is adjacent to my apartment building, so no matter what winter delivered, I've been able to travel underground and work out at least five days a week.

The club has also become my afternoon distraction. At times, my apartment feels claustrophobic, so I return with my laptop to an alternative, people-filled environment. And because, off-and-on, I've been a member for 30 years, I greet many old friends and meet new ones.

I've joined Chicago Sinai Congregation (walking distance) and attend weekly Torah study. Along with filling in the holes of my religious knowledge, membership has brought a sense of community and new friends.

I don't have to worry about home maintenance. When weather forecasters warned homeowners to beware of frozen pipes, icicles dangling from eaves, and sidewalks and driveways needing plowing, I was grateful I was no longer a homeowner.

<u>And now the cons:</u>

I have made only one friend in my building. In my old neighborhood, I knew nearly every family on my block. I had watched kids grow from babies to teens. In my apartment building, which is more like a dorm because of its thirty-something population, I have made only one good friend. She's the age of my daughters, and cares for me and makes me laugh just as my flesh-and-blood do.

I miss owning a dog. Although my building allows pets, and there are many I can coo at, including my friend's bity boy, I pine for a pup. But, the practical me understands I can't afford the extra expense, I'd have a hard time racing to a vet without a car, and potty breaks in a high rise are challenging.

I'm spending too much money.

I think it's a wash between my monthly rent and my former mortgage payment. And, with the absence of car expenses and lower utility bills, it would appear I'm in good financial shape.

But, with the pros I mentioned earlier, like my pricey health club and proximity to grocery shopping (Whole Foods) and department stores (Nordstrom's), I'm finding temptations hard to pass up. Thus, I'm wary every time I face a monthly statement.

Despite the cons I've confessed, I know that if I had stayed put, the traces of Tommy and our Golden Retriever, Buddy, would've trumped all and tinted my mood. I signed the lease; a new year, a new me.

QUE SERA, SERA

Anna goes to the kitchen to find scotch tape. She heads straight for a drawer and grabs a roll -- her Early Stage Alzheimer's hasn't yet robbed her of that discovery.

"How about here?" I ask. I am standing in the hallway of her home, at the foot of the staircase, holding up a lined page ripped from a notebook.

We selected this spot because anyone entering -- particularly her adult children and caregiver -- can't miss it. Anna hands me the tape and I affix the sign so it drops from a shelf to the right of the stairs. Dictated by my friend, it reads: IF I FORGET TO FEED MY CATS OR CHANGE THEIR LITTER, PLEASE DO SO.

"Thank you," she says to me, and we return to the couch where she spends her days adjacent to a small television. A table at arms length holds a large monthly calendar, the notebook, packages of gum, telephone numbers of her children, and various homeopathic medicines someone believes will help Anna snap out of her condition.

As evidenced by our sign, I am not in the alternative treatment camp. I've read up on Alzheimer's, and have the experience of caring for my husband, Tommy, whose dementia didn't lead to memory loss, but was equally unfixable. Instead of urging Anna to curb repetition, or pull herself out of depression, or halt her worries, I instead stick with wherever her slowly erasing mind lands.

Months ago, when Anna stopped remembering what she had done earlier the same day; I began to visit her weekly. As typical of those with the illness, she has no problem recalling episodes from long ago, and is delighted when I regularly recount our first meeting.

She perches on her couch, adjusts her two hearing aids -- which she says aren't working as they are supposed to -- and leans in for my story. "It was my first day in the exercise class," I say, using a slow cadence, as if it were a fairy tale. "You were in the first row near the mirror and I was in the back. You were dancing so gracefully, different than all of the others. I couldn't take my eyes off of you."

After class, I spotted Anna in the health club's lobby and stopped her to express my admiration. "I was a ballet dancer in my youth," she explained. "The movements are natural."

That meeting led to a deep friendship. I learned she was 10 years older than me, which brought me hope realizing I could possibly be in as great shape when I reached her milestone. She became an immediate fan of my memoir, "The Division Street Princess," and bought at least a dozen copies to give to friends. We were each other's cheerleaders.

On the couch, after the sign posting and our how-we-met story, Anna tells me, "I know how your husband Tommy must have felt. Like a prisoner." Although she declares this with each visit, I nod my head. "Que sera, sera," she says. "Whatever will be, will be. Remember that song? Doris Day, right?" She is proud she has made the right combination.

"Yes, it's from a movie," I say. "A classic Alfred Hitchcock."

I pull out my iPhone and find a clip of the scene in "The Man Who Knew Too Much" where Day is at the piano singing loudly so her son, who is trapped upstairs, can hear her. Jimmy Stewart is slinking out of the ballroom where the mini concert is being held.

Anna's eyes are giving her as much trouble as her ears, so she pulls my phone close to her face to discern the action and music. When the few minutes of play are completed, we sing together the lyrics. Her caregiver, Sonia, who is seated nearby, joins in.

Then, Anna rises from the couch, walks to the piano -- standing because I am seated on the chair that is usually at the instrument -- plays the tune, perfectly; by ear. I clap loudly, as if mirroring the movie star's volume.

In an hour, as I stand up to leave, Anna asks, "When are you coming back?" Her pencil is poised at the over-sized calendar.

"Sometime next week," I say, and step in for our usual hug and kiss. "I'll call you as soon as I get my schedule."

In he hallway I pass the taped sign and wonder if it will still be up when I return. "Que sera, sera," I think to myself, closing the door behind me. "Whatever will be, will be."

HOW JOURNALING PROPELS ME FORWARD

Every morning, after rising and making coffee, I sit on my couch with a 6" x 8" spiral notebook and a Pilot Razor Point Extra Fine pen.

For at least a half hour, I record a diary of what I did the day before, dreams and nightmares, wounds and applause, plus tasks due that day. As of this writing, I'm up to page 10,380.

While that number may sound impressive, it doesn't travel far enough back. I wish the innocent little girl I once was would have grabbed pen and paper as soon as she learned to print. If I had started then, writing my memoir, "The Division Street Princess," might have required less tunneling. To fill in, I had to rely on microfiche pages of Chicago newspapers, tales told by relatives, memories that had been bolted to my brain, and my imagination.

For my second book, a slight e-novel called, "She's Not The Type," I had some journal pages, but not the guts. The first half of that book is a roman a clef, somewhat based on my first marriage -- our secret romance, wedding, birth and upbringing of two daughters, and our eventual somber divorce after 30 years. The second half is pure fiction -- a wistful dream where the protagonist becomes a journalist and her mother, rather than dying young while in a pathetic second marriage, moves to Hawaii and finds true love.

In this current period of my life, with my morning journaling as sacred as a religious rite, I also read a page taken from past years. I do this because I want to learn my patterns -- worries that never came to pass, prophetic musings, and other buried gold.

Recently, I've been in 2012, reliving my husband Tommy's last weeks. Although my heart beats as I read about the emergency room visit when he became dehydrated, the astonishing discovery that it was throat cancer rather than dementia blocking his ability to swallow, ten harrowing days at Northwestern Memorial Hospital, and twelve at home in hospice, the most surprising take-away was my eerie calm.

When I discussed this odd composure with others who had experienced similar journeys, one friend said, "You did what you had to do." I'll accept that, but I have another theory: Because of my daily journaling and The Rookie Caregiver blog I was writing at the time, I had been able to release most of the shadows, fear, and grief.

Remarkably, on the entry I wrote November 4, 2012, just two days after Tommy died, I wrote: *Plan to start post for TRC about his death. Then, keep up until I have enough pages for a book. After that, get a fee for editing and self-publishing, do a cloud fundraising, and try to get book completed by May 2013. Goal.*

I'm a year late, but thanks to 112 backers on a Kickstarter campaign, it is happening. She Writes Press will publish "Green Nails and Other Acts of Rebellion: Life After Loss" September 2014.

It turns out it is not only starry-eyed goals that plump my journals, but other musings that bear repeating.

On November 9, 2012, one week after Tommy's death, I wrote: *Bank turned me down for a Home Equity Line of Credit, not enough income. Not surprised. Think I will eventually sell as house is way too big for one person & do I want hassle of roommates or borders? May be better for me to rent new apt. that can make my life easier and not have to depend on others. All options open.*

Those words turned into several posts on The Rookie Widow - a prophecy that took less time to accomplish than my third book. In a little over five months, I was settled into my new River North apartment.

Because I'm tech savvy, it's surprising I've resisted typing my daily words into a computer. But for me, there's something about pen and paper that better stirs my brain and soul. I'm grateful to journaling for buffing my writing voice, while also serving as memory chip, repository, therapist, best friend, cheerleader, and crystal ball. And coupled with that first cup of coffee in the morning -- for this writer, it has been the most nourishing way to start a new day.

CHEAPSKATE, ENVIRONMENTALIST, OR CHICKEN

I had my choice of a Ford Focus Hatchback or a Honda Insight Hybrid. Either would cost $47.04 for the four-hour rental I would use to drive to Old Orchard where I'd meet my friend, Ruth, for lunch.

This online search was prompted by the absence of my own Honda Fit, which I had returned to the leaseholder prior to moving downtown.

"Don't worry," I had told friends who worried the absence of a vehicle would curb my weekly visits. "I'll join a car-sharing service -- they're parked in my high-rise's garage -- so there won't be any interruption."

Immediately after unpacking, I signed up with Zipcar, paid a $60 annual membership fee, plus $9 per month for a complete damage waiver. But, in the 365 days I've had the plastic card in my wallet, I've never used it.

At first, I blamed my reluctance to the lack of available vehicles in my garage. Oh, there was a sampling several blocks away, but the trek eroded some of the ease I had envisioned.

Part of the problem is my four-feet-nine-inches and need for visibility. In order to lift me above the steering wheel, I must use two pillows. The thought of schlepping those booster seats to a far away car lot is unappealing.

My hesitation with Zipcar hasn't interrupted my promise to friends. Instead, I opt for the CTA, or Uber and Lyft ride-sharing apps with their private drivers.

But, with a one-and-a-half hour Purple Line Linden train to Central St. in Evanston, then a #201 bus to the shopping center on my calendar, I decided to finally reserve a car for the 16-mile trip. I'd still have to walk elsewhere to get a car, but I was willing.

As I perused my vehicle options, a trio of voices barged into my brain. First was the stingy sidekick. "If you take the train and bus, it'll only cost $2.50 round trip," she said, her demeanor mirroring a sensible accountant's. "Compare that to the $215.04 total with membership and renting. "

Then, another voice interrupted; this one with a righteous tone, "Well, I agree that ditching a car is smart, but more important than cost is the effect on the environment." She was the same noodge who berated me for leaving at home canvas bags when I shop at Whole Foods. "Air pollution, global warming," she droned.

The third voice chimed in -- timid, shaky. "Please don't drive," she said. "I'm scared. Remember what happened the last time, with the Prius and iGo?"

How could I forget? At the time, I was still living on the northwest side, and wanted to try car sharing before my move. With vehicles across the street in Independence Park, I thought it'd be a breeze.

But on the day of my experiment, no cars were available, so I walked nearly a mile to the nearest location. I followed instructions to unlock the door and start the ignition. I placed my two cushions on the driver's seat. Then, after lifting, stretching, and twisting to view the rear window, I slowly backed out.

I braked as I spotted a four-door parked at an angle just behind me. Was that a dent in its rear fender? My heart hammered; I started perspiring, I felt weak, faint. Had I already maimed a vehicle? Instead of exiting to find out, I continued on, still shaking but believing that if I interrupted my trial, I'd never gain the shared-ride experience. As soon as I arrived at my destination, I checked for damage on the Prius -- none. Then, I called iGo.

"I think I hit a parked car," I said, trembling as if I were confessing a murder. I provided all required information, then returned to the original lot. I took out my iPhone to capture the damage on the still-parked vehicle. But, I couldn't find any. The dent I had imagined was instead the fender's sloping design. I circled the car several times to make sure the two fenders matched. They did!

I called iGo again and reported my happy findings. "Great," the staffer said, "but we'll send you an accident report just in case." I filled it out and waited days, weeks, months, a year, but nothing more came of the incident. Still, it traumatized me. Ever since, I've been reluctant to drive an unfamiliar car.

So, I'll travel to Old Orchard via CTA. When Ruth praises my pluck, I'll tell her "saving money and the environment." But I'll confess to you: I'm a chicken -- a pint-sized hen that needs two booster seats to see over a steering wheel. Cluck. Cluck.

PLAYING THE FIELD

Five whites, two Blacks: three Jews, four Catholics. Not the first line of a joke that ends with, "walk into a bar," but the eclectic roster of men, over the age of 70, whom OurTime.com suggests are my matches.

Although I've often said I'm not eager to meet a new man -- either for companionship and especially not marriage -- it appears I lied, or changed my mind. Likely the latter, as I've been known to do that often in my roller coaster years.

Who needs a man? I would toss at my daughters or friends who wondered/worried at my inclination to cuddle with Netflix rather than seek a male in my widowed life.

Another excuse I have used for disdaining dating was that my second marriage to Tommy was so content, so stress-free (if you don't count the three years of caregiving before he died), that it'd likely be difficult to find someone as compatible as my dearly departed. "Low maintenance," was how I described him. And even when his aphasia and the trickling of dementia entered our union, he remained upbeat and sociable.

But now, as I'm attempting to confront a few items in my life that I realize are fear-based; i.e. swimming and driving an unfamiliar car, it hit me that dating is numero tres on the list. Because Our Time is targeted to older singles, I thought I'd give this virtual gang another go.

Fear of rejection certainly accompanies these searches, but fear of leaping into a relationship with the wrong guy is equally daunting. Because my two husbands sought after me, I didn't have to face rejection. My first, who I was married to for 30 years, chose me (until he didn't), and although I asked Tommy out for our first date, after that he wouldn't leave my side.

In between those two marriages, during my six years of singleness, I grabbed onto guys that any clear-eyed person could've seen were absolutely wrong for me. But in my pathetic neediness, I chose to refurbish their personalities and foibles until each one shined like a matinee idol.

I see a pattern in the romances I leapt into during that break: the men had an air of danger. Evidently, I had reverted to high school where the Tony's of my world triumphed over the Sheldon's. Ducktail haircuts, Lucky Strikes in their t-shirt pockets, ditching school; could anything have been more alluring to a good, little, Jewish girl?

My relationship with the adult bad boy I chose in the space between wedlocks lasted for several years. He was such an antidote to my rigid, silent first marriage that I batted away warning signs as if they were foam rubber baseballs. *So he drove too fast? So he smoked? So he smoked weed? So he channeled new age gurus? So his apartment was a mess? So he was a sloppy dresser? So he had intimate conversations with his harem of women friends?*

Get the picture? Eventually, it was the last *so* that ended the idyll. Despite all of the cons that mounted like a child's tower of blocks, I was still attached and jealous of his bond with his bevy of gals. When challenged, he chose them rather than me. I whimpered for a bit, then realized I had dodged a bullet. (But, he often visits me in my dreams, which I consider a safer habitat than real life.)

Now, in my current singleness, if I do receive responses from my Our Time United Nations, I'll likely reject some, and be rejected by others.

There may be dates involved; evenings that include uncomfortable high heels (me), dreaded auditions and boring biographies (both) -- all while my mind is zeroing in on his comb-over, toupee, paunch, age spots, or other blots. (He is likely doing the same when it is my turn to drone. *How can she be so short? Why does she tolerate those wrinkles? Hasn't she heard of hair dye?)*

I can handle those potential episodes. What I fear, I now realize, is that I haven't shucked enough neediness and am ripe for another wrong guy. Could a hunger for holding hands while strolling the river walk, or the scent of a freshly washed shirt while in a man's hug, and perhaps the chance to call someone "honey" shove me towards an unsuitable male?

Guess I'll have to risk it to find out.

ALL DRESSED UP AND...

Saturday, 5:20 p.m. In ten minutes I'd depart my apartment for the lobby where I'd use my cell phone to call Lyft for a pickup. My destination's address was memorized, ready to submit to the driver-- a Thai restaurant on Lawrence Ave. --where I'd meet, in person, a 77-year-old male from OurTime.com

Before this, I had stood before my bedroom's full-length mirror and surveyed my image: pricey black-and-white Eileen Fisher tank top and unconstructed grey jacket over black Gap jeans, black Stuart Weitzman strap sandals. I gave my outfit two thumbs up.

Along with my fashionable getup, I had enhanced my image by upgrading face and hair products. Instead of everyday Mac makeup, I used special occasion Sisley. Shampoo and conditioner got elevated, too. Kevin Murphy swapped for Bumble and bumble. The only part of my body that hadn't been creamed or painted was my nails. I hadn't had time for a professional manicure, so I removed chipped polish and applied a clear base coat. My bland nails would have to do.

Then, the phone rang.

"Just got in," said my date. "Can we postpone till seven?"

"No," I said, my voice level, but geared for a rise. "That's too late. I'm ready now. I'm all dressed and about to call a ride for the restaurant."

"I need to shower and change," he said, offering no reason or apology for the delay.

"What's the earliest you can make it?"

"6:30."

I'm thinking, *should've listened to my gut. In our first phone conversation, he had admitted he wasn't in contact with his adult kids; that's usually a red flag. He also divulged he was bounced from his job. Flag number two. Why had I even made a date with this loser?*

"Listen," I said, already angry with myself for using my overpriced cosmetics for a date that grew cloudier as the conversation continued. "You knew you had plans for six; you even confirmed the day before. You should have made it your business to be on time. This doesn't feel good. Let's forget about it."

"But, I have to clean up," he said. "You wouldn't want me to skip that." He was testy, as if I were the culprit.

"Goodbye," I said, stabbing the cell phone's red icon to end the call.

"Sorry," he got out before my line went dead.

All dressed up and nowhere to go, so I started dialing to seek an alternate dinner plan. "Oh, sorry," said my neighbor, Diane. "I'm going to Plum Market, but you're welcome to come along."

My friend Lisa responded, "Just got back in the house from gardening. Going to change and settle in. Any other time, I'd be on my way."

"About to get in the car for an event in the suburbs," said my ex-husband, who has remained a good friend. Sorry this happened to you."

"It's okay," I told each one. "I'm really happy to stay home. And, I'll have material for my blog. No great loss."

Resigned to my revised evening, and relieved I hadn't sprung for a manicure, I changed from my snazzy garb into decades-old leggings and t-shirt. I poured my usual thimble-full of chardonnay, placed a dinner tray on my lap and watched another episode of "The West Wing" and then the pilot of the British series of "House of Cards." Despite my face still in full makeup and my hair coiffed, I felt as settled and relaxed as a baby hippo in a puddle of soothing mud.

Putting the deleted date behind me, the next day I returned to scroll the dating site's latest matches. I had already met two other men, and although I didn't fall in love with either one, or they with me, they were nice, dependable, and stable.

The first two were Jewish (as was the dud), which sort of surprised me because I had chosen this site -- rather than the exclusive JDate -- so I could meet men of different races and religions.

But somehow I decided that selecting a member of my tribe moved the game along quicker, like a roll of the dice that allowed your token to skip several stops and land in a prime spot on the board.

Of course, every time I flipped past the Christians, I paused to muse. Tommy was gentile, and we had a compatible, loving 16-year-relationship and marriage. Why was I not willing to chance that again?

So now, I'll shift strategy. My last experience with a clansman has sent me back to ecumenism. This time, though, I'll heed my boundaries and only make plans with a man close to his kids and gainfully employed or retired.

I might even book a manicure.

PICK-UP LINES

"There's a kind of nice looking man at the pool. For you, not me. No ring. He's doing crosswords. What are you doing?"

"Thanks. On train home," I typed in response to Diane's text.

"Oh, perfect. Stop by."

In the next communiqué, instead of providing further description, my friend sent a photo of the man she was bagging. Evidently Diane took the shot surreptitiously because only half of his body was visible and a wooden fence obscured his image.

"Oh, a bit of a belly," she wrote. "But you're the only one who doesn't have one."

I had a second to enjoy her praise before this text arrived: "Crap, he's leaving. Scratch that. He just sat down under an umbrella. You'll walk into him. Facing snack bar."

How could I resist this summons, which was as tempting as a movie trailer promising love between two mature singles? In my version, and likely Diane's, the hilarious sidekick plays a major role in bringing the widow and widower (preferably for pathos) together.

With conjured music guiding my path -- think trumpets -- I took the elevator to the fourth floor of our health club, and then paused to survey the scene. Row upon row of brown weaved lounge chairs spread out on a deck that seemed the size of a football field. A crowd, out of central casting, occupied most: they were young -- 20's and 30's; the men handsome and sculpted, the women, tall, thin with long blonde or brunette hair and wearing bikinis as bity as a baby's first swimsuit. (Trumpets give way to cellos.)

Fortunately, I was fully clothed, so there was no need to contrast my shape -- which does indeed include a belly -- against the slender panorama mocking my age, height, wrinkled skin, and hidden middle.

With Diane's treasure map in mind, I easily spotted our quarry. He was sort of heavy set, grey hair, likely my age, probably Jewish (could be Greek or Italian), definitely someone I would've graced with a second glance had I spotted him on my own.

I looked at him; he looked at me. I continued my walk.

"So, what do you think?" Diane asked. I pulled up a chair, and then dropped my backpack on the concrete, and me in the seat.

"He looks okay," I said. Actually, he was my body type. I never minded a bit of zaftig-ness because the shape reminded me of my beloved dad. (In Tommy's case, although he was svelte and toned, I relented because my dearest made up for it with his adoration.)

"You must be thirsty," Diane said, offering a hand to tug me out of the chair. "Let's go back to the snack bar and get you some water."

Obviously, she was rehearsing her own lines for our upcoming film and intent on moving the scene along. I worried: for comic effect, would she elbow me onto his lap?

The man, wait, let's give him a name: Larry, was still seated in his lounge chair. We took note again of his absence of a ring or a female companion. En route, with the sun stewing my covered body, I again viewed the guys and gals. I overheard these pick-up lines: *Didn't you go to Madison? You were in my MBA program, right?*

Best pal sidekick and I did our trip, and on the reverse, I looked at him, he looked at me. Then, our detective duo returned to our chairs. "Now, go up and talk to him," Diane said.

"What would I say?"

"You're clever; you can think of something."

"How about a mistaken identity ploy?" I said. *Hi, Larry, I thought you looked familiar. Didn't we meet at Hedy and Mort's party?*

I was clever. By starting out with a name, he'd have to respond with his real one. And by using a popular couple that are my friends, and who host many events, perhaps we had met at one of their occasions.

"That'll work," Diane said.

"Or, I could just try, *Hi, I noticed you're not wearing a wedding ring and you're alone. You appear to be in my age group and my preferred body type. I'm a widow on the hunt. May I sit down and chat?*

"That would work, too," she said.

"What if he doesn't speak English? Then what?"

"Better yet," she said. "Haven't you seen movies where the language barrier is conquered by the language of love?"

We tested a few more pick-up lines as I gained courage. But, by the time we settled on the mistaken identity ploy, Larry was gone.

Sigh. Broken up before first date. Cue the violins.

TOMMY HAS BOUNDARIES

An email from Our Time, the online dating site, alerted me to a new message: "How about 2 p.m. at Meinle, the coffee shop at Addison and Southport?"

I was pleased to see these details from my latest match. In an earlier email, I told him I was going to be on Southport for a 3:30 movie at the Music Box, and since he revealed he lived near Lakeview High School, I gave him the option of naming a place for our first meeting.

"Sounds good," I wrote back. Then, "I'm going to take a chance and give you my real name and phone number."

I was aware this was a risk, but our previous messages signaled a safe bet. In those, I learned he was a former journalist and PR guy, kept fit, was divorced, traveled, and had two kids. On paper, he deserved a look-see.

I added: "I'd also appreciate <u>your</u> contact information. This way, we can do background checks and text if there are delays or cold feet."

A few hours passed as I prepared my wardrobe and kept busy with tasks to prevent obsessing about the meeting. Although I had had several dates with Our Time matches, and they turned out pleasant and interesting, I still became anxious about initial sightings. Those opening minutes always felt to me like a Broadway audition, where I'm probably all-wrong for the part.

Soon it would be time to get dressed for my 2 p.m. coffee date, but I hadn't yet heard from Match6. Now I had a dilemma: Did he not read my online email requesting his contact information and would just show up at Meinle?

Or, had he read it, done due diligence to check me out and learn that I frequently write about my dates. Did that scare him off? Then, the phone rang. It was a 773 area code, but no caller I.D. It could've been a marketer, but I decided to answer it.

"Hello, is this Elaine?" From the sound of his voice, I knew I'd be exchanging my date wardrobe for everyday clothes.

"I know who you are," he said. "We've met. Tommy and I worked out at the Y together. He used to bring me his old golf magazines. Remember, I'd run into the two of you at Dapper's diner? Tommy introduced us; I remember you being nice."

Match6 told me his real name and I tried to picture him and place him in the setting he revealed. I couldn't get a sharp image, but think he was tall and good-looking. Despite his compliment, I knew our date was in jeopardy.

"I don't feel comfortable," he said. "I hope you understand. It's a little too close to home."

"Of course I understand," I said, but thought: S**t! Why did I give him my real name? If I had waited for our meeting to exchange details, Match6 might have thought me appealing enough to give loyalty a pass.

"Maybe we'll get together at some point," he said. "Trade war stories about online dating."

"That'd be great," I said, knowing it wouldn't happen.

With time on my hands, I pondered why I had sabotaged myself by prematurely revealing my identity. Soon enough, I felt a tap on my shoulder. It was my dearly departed, moving in my imagination from the past tense to the present.

"Hi Wifey," he said. Tommy was smiling, devilishly. "How's your dating life going?"

"It was you, Hubber, wasn't it? You put the idea in my head to out myself. You knew Match6 would look me up and get cold feet."

"I'm not confessing to anything," Tommy said. His smile grew broader and soon he was laughing.

It was wonderful to envision him joyous, but then I sobered. "Why didn't you want me to meet him? We could've had a date. Not marriage, as I've often promised, but a companion."

"Listen sweetheart," he said. "I know you're trying to find a boyfriend, but I have boundaries. The guy is my friend, off limits. It'll be easier for me if your fella is a stranger."

"OK," I said. "No one in your circle. No Y or golf buddies."

So, on my list of criteria for potential dates -- which already included "must love animals, be connected to his children, be under the age of 85" -- I added, "no one who's a pal of Tommy."

With that, I felt a soft kiss on my cheek. Then, my Hubber was gone.

FULL DISCLOSURE

I got weary of all the peppy profile suggestions from online dating sites, which go something like this: *What makes you happy? What do you most enjoy doing? What are some things you can't live without?* Their upbeat eagerness -- likely penned by 20-somethings or techies in India -- was beginning to rile me.

So on my latest attempt, on a site called JPe*pleMeet.com (the asterisk is subbing for a Star of David, just in case you weren't hip to what "J" stands for), I decided to experiment and swipe starry-eyed for wry, impolite, and honest. Then, see if anyone would bite.

In the paragraph that asks for "A little about me..." I wrote:

"Full disclosure: I'm an early riser and fade in the afternoons. I exercise regularly but need someone to open jar lids. I gave up my car when moving downtown, so if you still drive, including "at night," you're my hero. Sorry if you're down in the dumps, but I'm looking for someone upbeat. You should be able to text.

"Please have a smart phone and know how to send messages. I love quality TV. If you haven't heard of Netflix, we're likely not a match. And if you don't have a sense of humor, we have nothing in common."

Also, in this third dating site that I've visited -- JDate and Our Time are the other two -- I made my desired age range 70 to 80, and location, Chicago. Despite my specified criterion, you can bet I'll get responses from 65-year-olds living in Denver, or 87-year-olds that "Like" my profile. Proof to me that most men don't read any of the physical descriptions beyond "athletic and toned." (Some jerks go so far as to warn us women not to message if we're overweight.)

While my "A little about me..." is on target, I omitted some other truths. But at some point, when I truly get burnt-out on these virtual experiences, I'll add: "I go to bed at 8 p.m., so if you're seeking a dance partner or a party girl, step away from the screen. I have a short attention span. If our lunch date lasts longer than one-and-a-half hours, I'll make an excuse to depart. It will either be boredom that sends me scurrying, or a need for an afternoon nap."

Based on my above bitchiness, you might assume I've had dreadful experiences with online dates. Au contraire. Through Our Time, I've gone out on four lunch and two dinner dates with quite pleasant men. They were all nice looking, well-dressed, smart, stable, sane, and impressively, all picked up the check for my meal.

Here's a little about them. But instead of disclosing their screen names, I'll call them by my labels.

The Libertarian was 72, possibly a hippie in his youth, and lived in a beautiful, homey condo overlooking Millennium Park. We had dinner at an Asian restaurant, and afterwards went to his place so I could attempt to set up his Apple TV. No hanky panky, and no spark for either of us. But we are Facebook friends.

I had two dates with the Chef, 85. The first was lunch at Gene & Georgetti's, and the second was a gourmet dinner at his luxurious condo. Both of us were very staid, the only heartbeats were for his cooking.

At 82, Mr. Fox Valley was a genial caregiver and widower. He was intrigued enough to drive the 30-or so miles to meet me for lunch in my neighborhood. He invited me to spend a weekend at his home, but when I froze, he quickly added, "I have two bedrooms." I considered a day trip, but after contemplating the folly of a city-to-whistle-stop relationship, I backed out. We remain friends.

The Professor was date number four, 72, a widower from Evanston. We met halfway at Cafe Selmarie in Lincoln Square. We talked ill spouses and bad deaths, computers, and families. We each expressed "had a nice time." I'm not sure who will make the next move.

Knowing you, dear reader, you're already combing my descriptions for your favorite and wondering why romance hasn't swooped up and blinded us. I have a theory: For the men, they're likely being pursued by a gaggle of grandmas and are taking their time to enjoy the attention and dates.

As for me, if you've read between the lines of "A little about me..." you'll see a very ambivalent dater who enjoys writing about matchmaking more than actually doing it. And then there's this: None were Tommy.

CALIFORNIA DREAMING, PART TWO

I was perched on a stool at the bar of Intelligentsia, a coffee shop on East Randolph St. in Chicago. While I waited for my decaf to be brewed, I pulled out a notebook that I had recently purchased in Los Angeles at Muji, a hip Japanese retailer that sells clothing, furniture, and stationary.

While my small ritual was taking place in the city of my birth, and where I have lived for a majority of my 75 years, my mind travelled to the Intelligentsia on Silver Lake Blvd., in Los Angeles, where my daughter, Jill, and her family live. Both the shop, and the notebook -- which was opened to a blank page -- seemed to be omens of a possible new future.

It all started a few weeks ago on a four-day trip. My 17-year-old grandson, Isaac, and I were seated at Sqirl, a breakfast spot in East Hollywood. I was eating "Crispy Kokuho Rose Brown Rice Salad, Lemongrass, Mint, Cilantro, Ginger with a fried egg," while Isaac chose the Sweet side of the menu, "Brioche Toast with Guittard Chocolate Ganache, Nut Butter, and Fleur De Sel."

My fashionable grandson had selected Muji and Sqirl for a morning we were spending together. I was relishing his company -- and wasn't even miffed when he recoiled as I combined our leftovers into one take-home container.

"Grandma, you can't do that!" he said, as he watched me place the egg concoction and sugary bread in a Styrofoam nest. Isaac looked appalled, as if I were a peasant who had wandered into this chic spot.

"I can't leave them behind," I said. "Besides, you don't want your brioche, and I'll be eating both of them."

"Use two boxes!" he said, and closed his eyes at his gauche grandmother.

Isaac shook his head and didn't press it further, but our affectionate repartee made me realize how much I missed him and the rest of his family. And during that particular visit to L.A., I not only got to see Jill's crew, but also my other daughter, Faith, and my 12-year-old granddaughter, Betsy, who were visiting from Boston.

For me, those four days on the West Coast were precious, something to be savored as much as my meal.

Isaac must've felt a similar tug, because during our walk to his car, he said, "Grandma, why don't you move here?"

"I did consider it last year," I told him, "then chickened out. Maybe this time I'll experiment, rent a place for a few weeks and see how it feels to live here independently."

He brightened. "That sounds like a good plan."

And with those words, wheels began to spin. "I'll come for the whole month of February," I told Jill. "Rent an Airbnb that'll be walking distance to your house. This way, I'll miss part of Chicago's horrible winter."

Both of us went on the website where people lease their spare rooms, coach houses, or furnished apartments. "Here's one just seven minutes from me," Jill said, in an email that accompanied a neighborhood map.

Although other L.A. sections would likely house people nearer my age, I like Silver Lake because it's similar to Chicago's Wicker Park -- with restaurants and boutiques in easy walking distance. Any eventual move wouldn't make sense if I couldn't easily trot over to Jill's, or to Intelligentsia.

After I researched her pick and was about to book it, another communiqué came from my co-conspirator. "Why wait until February?" she said. "Come sooner."

"How about two weeks in November, with Thanksgiving included?" I said. "The holidays are hard without family."

Jill gave the idea her blessing. And then the experiment seemed to morph into something more permanent, with each of us positing advantages: "I've already downsized," I said. "It'd be one truck load going cross country."

Then, "If I lived close enough and you get delayed at work, I could go over and start dinner."

"You're an early riser," Jill said, warming to the concept. "I can sleep in and you can come over in the morning to start Felix's breakfast." The image of my 5-year-old grandson's sleep-tussled head upped the ante.

So is it Chicago's past brutal winter that sparked this second, more serious pull to sunny California? Or, is it the realization that the luscious visit with Isaac and his family could be repeated weekly, rather than three times a year?

And maybe Faith and Betsy would move to L.A.? Perhaps my Chicago friends would be frequent visitors? Maybe I'll adopt a dog, lease a Honda? Oh, there's no end to positive scenarios I can dream up.

TOMMY INTERVENES

"Why wasn't I consulted?"

"You're dead; you don't get a vote."

My late husband had taken advantage of my middle-of-the-night bathroom break to jump in the empty half of my bed. It was just enough time to rouse me from sleep and to get him chatty.

"Since I live in your head, you're taking me with you, right? Whether I like it or not."

"It's an experiment, sweetheart," I said. "Two weeks, in an apartment separate from Jilly, to see if I can live independently in L.A."

"I never liked L.A."

"That's because we didn't drive on our visits; you hated being stuck in her house while I clung to my grandkids."

"So, are you really going to drive in L.A? I read on your blog that you might lease a Honda?"

I paused on the dialog bouncing in my brain. *Honda.* Did that vehicle stir unpleasant memories for my deceased husband? Was he still rankled because I took away his car keys when his illness made it unsafe for him to drive?"

If so, he didn't bring it up, but went on to say, "The hills in Silver Lake, the 110? Are you prepared to deal with those?"

Boy, my hubby of 14 years sure knew my tender spots. Had he picked up on my own anxiety as I boldly wrote my intent to be a driver in L.A.?

"And, 'adopt a dog'? You sure know how to hurt a guy. I thought we decided that after Buddy died, we wouldn't get another. Too expensive, too much potential for heartbreak. Weren't those your words?"

"I was only daydreaming," I said. "My readers like upbeat. If I had admitted my fears or hesitations, I'd lose the readers who count on my positivity."

"So, why bring me into this conversation that you're surely going to write about?" he said. "Talking to your dead husband isn't a ray of sunshine."

"You're wrong. My readers love it when I bring you back. It lets them know, that with a little imagination, they can resurrect their dearly departed."

"Glad I can be of service."

"So, are you mollified, sweetheart?"

"One more thing," he said. "If my numbers are correct, this would be your sixteenth move since 1960 and your first marriage. Right?"

I paused to count, and as I did a slideshow glided past my closed eyes.

See the walk-up apartment in Rogers Park, one- and two-bedroom apartments in Prairie Shores, captain's quarters in Massachusetts, a Glenview bi-level, a South Commons townhouse, condos in Streeterville and Michigan Ave., an Old Town rehab, a West town loft, a Lakeview townhouse, a Dakin Street single family, and now, a River North rental.

Each image carried its own emotional high- and low-points. There's the bright-eyed newly married couple. Two giggly girls born 18 months apart. Feeling fish-out-of-water in suburban and country homes. A surprise divorce. A happy remarriage. Shocking death. Resilient widowhood.

"Seventeen," I said, correcting his math.

Instead of judging, he said, "Remember I told you I'd only leave Dakin Street feet first?"

"You kept your word."

"But, here I am, with you in a high-rise, where I never wanted to be."

"Couldn't stay away? Miss me as much as I miss you?"

"Of course. And, I saw you during Chicago's last winter. I was relieved you weren't still in our house dealing with icy sidewalks, frozen pipes, and a snowbound garage."

"So, along with me being able to see much more of my family, you can appreciate the advantages of sunny California." I said. "Golf for you, year-round."

"Sweetheart," he said. "Up here, we not only have golf year-round, but also twenty-four seven, no green fees, no reservations, and never a foursome ahead. Why do you think it's called Heaven?"

"Okay, honey," I said. "I apologize for not consulting you sooner. So what's your verdict about a possible number seventeen?"

There was a pause, then this: "I see that the Tommy Bahama clothing store has some cool golf shirts. Can you pack me a few?"

"Done," I said. And with that last word, I drifted off to sleep. The image of my hubber garbed in a colorful, Hawaiian shirt, golf club aloft, and his Cubs baseball cap shielding his brown eyes from the California sun was as soothing as a lullaby.

UNTETHERED

I have no husband, no house, no dog, no car and no debt. For the first time in years, I am untethered. When that thought bore into my brain, I had a light-bulb moment. Instead of a two-week experiment of living independently in Los Angeles, as I had originally planned, why not jump in and find a one-year rental?

"I'll sublet my apartment and avoid paying rent on two places and on a round-trip flight," I said in a text to my daughter, Jill. And as I did tiny typing, I felt as euphoric as if I had just come up with a cure for a confounding disease.

When I posited this same untethered and economic reasoning to neighbors, friends, and relatives -- who have been privy to swift decisions and moves in my past -- they responded with either thumbs up or down.

"I'm 76 and currently in good health," I pressed on, hoping to swat away debate. "If I'm going to make a major move, it should be sooner rather than later. I don't want to wait until my daughters are touring nursing homes for their dear old mum."

And despite my assurances that previous hasty steps have always landed me on my feet, I could imagine my worriers trembling, as if I were about to skydive and they were watching helpless from the ground below.

It didn't take long for Jill to respond to my text. "Whoa," she sent back. "Take the expense out of the equation. Instead of moving here, what about extending the two weeks to an entire month? See how it feels to drive our hills, and to experience everyday life here?

"It's your anxiety that has you speeding ahead," she diagnosed. Jill has previously identified this condition, but after her text, I wondered: could she be having second thoughts about my slide from third base in Chicago to Home in L.A.?

I took the preemptive route. "If you're concerned that I'll turn into a crone [Wikipedia: disagreeable, malicious, or sinister in manner, often with magical or supernatural associations that can make her either helpful or obstructing], you needn't worry. When I can see you year 'round, rather than three times a year, I won't be so demanding of your time."

"I'm not worried," she said.

But am I? I accepted Jill's suggestion. Instead of rushing ahead, I will book the entire month of November in Los Angeles as a test drive. Accompanying my excitement, though, is a new internal query: How will I spend the 30 days to prevent becoming a drain on my daughter and her family?

To answer, I perused my August calendar.

Penciled in are lunches with friends, a haircut, a therapy appointment, a Mani/Pedi, doctor and dentist visits, workouts at a health club, a party, Saturday Torah study, and client meetings. November already has two major scheduled dates: a reading for my new memoir in Los Angeles at Skylight Books on the 19th and Thanksgiving on the 27th, which gives me a head start.

So, prior to November, I will seek surrogates for many of the above engagements. Along with these out-of-the-house appointments, I'll have my journal and laptop for daily writing, and several books that have been twiddling their pages on my nightstand.

"Whatever you find," I told Jill who is spearheading the November house search, "it must have a deck so I can sit outside with my morning coffee and notebook." This is the image I draw into my brain at 2:30 a.m., when excitement or anxiety (is the kid right?) jiggles me out of slumber.

In an effort to lull myself back to sleep, I take three deep breaths; hold each for a moment, and then release -- just as instructed in my daily relaxation podcast. And, as each part of my body is coaxed to soften, I conjure a still-dark morning in Los Angeles, a deck chair, side table, a cup of tongue-burning Intelligentsia coffee, my journal, and my Extra Fine Razor Point Pilot Pen.

Like a dog with an eager nose (If a permanent move is in my future, I will have a rescued pup at my side.), I sniff the air to catch scents of nearby blossoms and fruit trees. It is early, pre-dawn; no one else is awake. A porch light illuminates my writing. There is no noise, save indigenous birds that chirp me a "good morning."

This image -- serene and soulful -- is embedded in my brain. If any of my fretting friends posit, "what if's," or if my own quivering surfaces, I'll just take my three deep breaths, and as I exhale, replay my imagined scene. I can almost smell the peach trees, can't you?

MATCHMAKER, MATCHMAKER

Our Time is super excited. "You have 110 new profile views and 15 new messages!" it writes, as enthusiastic as a prospector finding gold.

Although weeks earlier I had dropped my membership and checked "do not automatically renew," the online dating site continues to send me these cheery emails. I imagine it -- and JDate, another of my experiments -- somewhere in cyberspace clucking at my resistance.

"What's her problem?" I hear the OT yenta say. (Naturally, if I were going to use my imagination to conjure my pesterers, they wouldn't be coders using algorithms to find me a match. In my zany brain, the two sites are women wearing babushkas, like old-world matchmakers eager to arrange a *shidduch* between two lonely singles.)

"She thinks she's so high and mighty," sniffs the JDate version. "I fixed her up with four eligibles, each one a mensch, and did she appreciate? *Vadyathink?"* (Excuse the ethnic patter; but, I'm Jewish so it's allowed. Also, I can't seem to stop.)

Now, here's where my imagination takes another leap. Although these two figments are in cyberspace, and my mother, Min, is in heaven, I figure she can't resist getting in on a conversation where her daughter is the topic.

"Don't look at me," she says. "I tried, told her to be sexier and younger in her profile. But, did she listen to me? It's just like when she was a teenager and...."

"Min," the yentas interrupt. Evidently, they have easily accepted photo-shopping her into the picture and chat. "Please stick to the subject. It's the present day. Your 76-year-old daughter, who is not getting any younger, is the one we're trying to fix up. Forget about the past."

With that, and without validation for her vote, Mom fades out and we're left with OT and JDate.

"Obviously, we're using the wrong approach," OT says to JDate. "She's not buying our daily e-mails. She knows that if she clicks on them, she'll be asked to rejoin."

"We can't let her get away," JDate says. "We don't want to see our CityGirl go through life without a man."

OT laughs. "She was CityGirl with you? Hah! She was Tiny75 with me."

I allowed this silly scenario to enter my brain because I was also wondering why I had put the brakes on my search for a significant other. As the yentas indicated, I did go on dates with four eligible, honest, and wholesome males. Although sparks didn't ignite, based on this positive experience, why didn't I continue to seek a match?

The answer: I found another passion, one as all consuming, thrilling, and with the possibility of a life-changing outcome. If you are a steady reader of this blog (a *shonda* if you are not), you're up to speed on my decision to test-drive Los Angeles in November for a possible move to that city.

This current project contains all of the delicious elements I require. It: 1) alleviates boredom, 2) allows me to make a checklist, 3) encourages research; i.e. synagogues, civic groups, salons, and therapists, and 4) entertains friends and relatives who vicariously join in on my flights of fancy.

"She's delusional." It's one half of the matchmaking pair intruding on my rationale. "You know once Tiny75 gets to L.A., and sets everything up, I predict that within a year, she's going to need another challenge."

"Oh, you're so right," says JDate. "And then she'll write about it, just like she did about our sites, mocking our sincere desire to link pathetic singles."

"You know, I've often wondered if the only reason CityGirl visited us was to get story ideas," OT says. "I feel so used."

"There is some consolation," JDate continues. "She'll start writing about L.A. and although the first few blog posts will be rah-rah -- the sunshine, her new friends, her family..."

OT interrupted. "Oy, be prepared for her glowing reviews of her grandchildren. How smart! How handsome! How polite! I don't know if I can take it."

"But knowing Tiny75 -- who will soon be Sun-Wrinkled76 -- we won't have to wait long for her beefs to surface."

JDate erupts in giggles. Soon she is rollicking. "She'll be slamming the tall and skinny starlets sipping their lattes at her precious Intelligentsia."

"What about the 20-somethings working on their screenplays? I can't wait to read her critiques of them!"

"Hold on a minute," JDate says. "Those writers are likely to be Jewish, right? Maybe a few will have widowed grandfathers to match with our old girl? What could entice her back into the fold."

"'Still drives' always works," OT says. "And, if we throw in 'at night;' she's hooked."

WALKING DISTANCE

In 1981, my first husband and I, and our two daughters, were living in a townhouse on N. LaSalle St. in Chicago. Our zip code was 60610.

My mother Min liked our location; so with my encouragement, she submitted an application to move her and her second husband into a senior citizen building that was walking distance from my home.

In December of that same year, as relatives and friends sat somberly in our living room with its vaulted ceiling that rose two floors up, I told of Mom's plans to those who had gathered for her *Shiva.* "She was so excited that she'd be living close to the kids and me," I said, "but it wasn't to be." The mourners nodded their heads and wiped away tears.

Through all of my essays about possibly moving to Los Angeles to be walking distance to my daughter Jill and her family, I hadn't thought about this long-ago scene.

But now, when I recall my mother's untimely death from a heart attack at 67, the line that reverberates is this: *I never got a chance to tell her how I felt; to mend things with her.*

If you've read my first memoir, "The Division Street Princess," you're aware I spent most of my childhood, and a good deal of adulthood, hoping to persuade Mom to love me for the person I truly was. And more importantly, to overcome my feeling that she was disappointed I wasn't taller, slimmer, and prettier.

When my aunts -- her sisters -- read my book, they were shocked to learn my dim assessment of the relationship. "Your mother loved you. She was so proud of you. How could you believe otherwise?"

But, our <u>own</u> truth often veers from what others perceive. And while her sisters likely heard Mom *kvelling* about me, I instead stored these childhood directives: Stand up straight. Comb your hair. You don't need that cake, and other orders that seem innocuous now. How could those words wound me so? Why have I carried them, like backpacks filled with rocks instead of school supplies, all these years?

Although Mother never made it to the apartment down the block from me, I may get to move across the country to a rental walking distance to Jill. And, if my other daughter, Faith, is fortunate enough to win another months-long writing assignment in L.A., my firstborn and me could possibly be roommates or neighbors.

To ease a potential departure from a city I have lived in nearly my entire life, and from dear friends and relatives, I'm considering the move a gift and opportunity -- which I never got with Min -- to assure there are no scenes or stings left over from my daughters' childhoods that <u>they</u> lug, or drop on a therapist's couch. And although I believe, and you likely do, too, that my daughters and I have an enviable and uncommon bond, do we really know their truths? Consider how divergent my aunts' opinions were from mine.

And perhaps my mother had her own wounds, inflicted by angelic me, that she kept hidden. What a pity it was that we -- who believed we had all the time in the world -- missed out on having conversations that surely would've resulted in hugs and vows.

Along with this late-in-life desire, to be a blame-free mother to my daughters, the other tasks to be addressed in a relocation would be:

To be a better grandmother and mother-in-law, and friend to Jill's *machetunim* (my son-in-law's parents), and to first cousins living in Beverly Hills. Then there's the crowd of former Chicagoans and current Los Angelinos whom I hope to reconnect with.

This goal -- likely prompted by my recently attaining the age of 76 -- is partially based on a belief that I may have come up short with this far-away group. I could blame it on distance, but it also could be that I lack a certain keep-in-touch gene.

But, it's not too late to improve my mother/grandmother/in-law/cousin/friend relationships. Proximity will help. Desire on my part will certainly up my chances. And, willingness by those on the other side will guarantee it.

So, dearest mother Min, I deeply regret we never had that chance to live in homes walking distance from one another, and to smooth over wrinkles that foolishly left me wanting. Now, I've been offered an opening with my own kin. I hope to take it.

LEAVING HOME

The voice was familiar, but I was having trouble placing it. In past conversations that occurred in my head, the participants were deceased, but still chatty. There were talks with my husband, Tommy, and with my parents, Min and Irv. While all of these episodes were tinged with the sadness of loss, I relished my brain's ability to bring these characters back to life, even if briefly.

I was narrowing in on identifying my imagination's latest speaker: it was a woman's voice, young, and definitely not coming from the afterlife. When she continued talking, I felt as happy as if I were welcoming home a long-lost relative.

"I know that emotion you're feeling," she said. "It was the same one we experienced in other parts of our lives. Think back."

She was my 25-year-old self who had evidently decided to reappear at a critical juncture in my journey. How odd that a youngster like that felt it necessary to counsel the 76-year-old she had become. But, I was delighted to see her. I took a moment to bring her full force into my vision: her brunette hair, her pretty green eyes covered by dark-framed glasses, her sweetheart-shaped face, and her welcoming smile.

I patted the empty side of my bed, inviting young Elaine to take a comfy place next to me. She slid in and I sighed as I took note of the extra inches of height awarded to the younger me. "What brings you here?" I said.

"Well, I could see you struggling with your decision to leave Chicago for Los Angeles. I watched you tossing each night, and wrestling with second thoughts. It was painful for me to witness that, so I thought it wise to reappear and help you out."

"It's not really second thoughts," I told this cutie pie sharing my bed. "I know I want to be closer to my daughters, and it's important to do it now, when I'm untethered and in good health. But after I enjoyed lunches and dinners with close friends, I felt sad, and wondered how I'd get along without these people in my day-to-day life."

"Yeah, I saw that," she said, "and I felt your sadness. You may not remember, but you've experienced the same emotion several times over the years. It's called 'separation anxiety.'"

"Hmm," I said, "that's interesting. I thought it was the separation from my daughters that was pulling me towards the West Coast. Now you're telling me the same feeling is tugging me back?"

"Think 1963," she said, pausing a moment for me to envision calendar pages flipping to that year. 'Your -- or should I say 'our' -- first husband was called up to serve in Fort Devens, Mass., and you accompanied him. Remember how you cried at the thought of leaving your mother behind? Separation, sweetheart, separation."

So that's why it was my 25-year-old self who had volunteered for this lecture. She was present. Married just three years earlier, leaving the home she shared with her widowed mother. No wonder she felt so vulnerable.

"I have another," I said, grateful I could contribute to our memory bank. "There was the time when he and I left our daughters behind with sitters and travelled to London. We were supposed to stay for two weeks, but I missed the girls so much, I insisted we return after one week."

"Separation," she repeated, "separation. You felt it with Faith and Jill when they were toddlers and you've continued to have a hard time with their absence. But the important thing to remember, dearest, is that these feelings are natural; they're what make us human. We love, and become attached to people, and we feel pain when we leave them."

"Another thing to keep in mind," said my guru "is that in those earlier experiences, you didn't lose the people you left behind. When you moved to Massachusetts, and said goodbye to your mother and best friend, you phoned them regularly. This time, along with calls, Skypes, email and Facebook, you can periodically fly back to Chicago for reunions with special pals."

"Thanks, sweetheart," I said, "You've really made me feel better. Is there anything I can do for you?"

Young Elaine contemplated my question, and then said, "I do have one request." She grabbed my hand as if to insure my attention.

"Don't let separation anxiety interrupt forward moves. I -- and all of your younger selves -- would be so bored if you suddenly decided to just stay put."

I gave our clasped hands a shake, kissed her adorable forehead, and then turned over to sleep peacefully the rest of the night.

MY MAGIC ACT

Anthony is six-five, nearly two feet taller than I. But as he steps into my Lilliputian-sized apartment, he does not seem to be dismayed by the ceilings he can likely touch on tip toes with an outstretched arm, or the walls he can reach a few feet away in either direction.

In fact, this young man seems pleased at the condition of my place and the scenic view from my expansive windows. But when I reveal the bedroom, which is concealed behind a sliding door, he folds his arms and says, "I'll have to switch out the bed for king-size."

"That's a shame," I tell him, "it's only a year-and-a-half old." We both stare at the full-size box spring and mattress, with Anthony envisioning how to fit in a new larger one. As for me, I'm conjuring the one I left behind when I moved from the Dakin St. house I shared with Tommy, to this River North high rise.

In that transition, I used an estate sale to dispose of most of my furniture and the contents of closets, drawers, shelves, and cupboards. Poof; 14 years of marital accumulation gone, as if a magician had waved a wand, making all disappear -except for memories.

With my upcoming move from Chicago to Los Angeles, I am the sorcerer. Faster than you can say "abracadabra," via a Craigslist ad, I found Anthony to take over the remaining six months of my lease, thus avoiding a two-month penalty. The slight-of-hand I used to lure him simply involved accepting the suggestion of my designer friend, Karen, and changing the listing from "rental" to "furnished-rental."

"A cross-country moving truck would be too expensive," I explained to those still reeling from my announcement that I not only decided to move to L.A., but it would take place in one month's time.

Of course, Anthony isn't concerned with my logic; he had been seeking a temporary residence until a nearby condo he is rehabbing is finished, so our quick-change act works out well for both of us.

When we turn to study my mini office with the sapphire blue desk and bench, Anthony laughs as I say, "you'll never fit there."

My friend Chris, an artist, not only painted the two pieces a bright color to disguise their country-style provenance, but he cut the legs to make it fit my four-nine size.

That same blue color transformed our coffee table -- the one that stood between Tommy's and my facing couches, home for the pencils he used for his cross-word puzzles, TV remotes, and the Post-it notes that conveyed our chatter in the last silent years of his life.

In this downtown apartment, the table has held the same props, except for the crossword puzzles. Now, the Post-it notes are only used for reminders from my buzzing brain.

In that previous move in April 2013, I stood at the living room window early in the morning awaiting the arrival of the truck that would cart away my small load. This time, there will be no window watching for I am using a large grocery cart to transport boxes to a USP store two blocks away. Cartons of photographs, previously stored in garages, or basements, lockers, and closets have already gone to my daughter Jill's home in Los Angeles.

"Do you want my china?" I asked in a text to her. Six dinner-sized and six salad-sized Wedgewood were rescued from the set I had left for the house sale. I've had them for 54 years, 24 longer than the marriage that brought them.

"Nah," was Jill's first response to my offer. Then this, "I think I do want those dishes. Yom Kippur realization!" (Some spiritualism at play here?)

Recently, my ex-spouse came to my apartment to pick up a scarf she had left behind at an event we both attended. Because I was in that neighborhood for a lunch date, I was able to retrieve it for her. "How can you leave all of this behind?" she said, her eyes tearing as she scanned the space.

"It's just stuff," I said.

"But, you did such a great job putting it all together."

Later, my therapist suggested that what my former spouse really meant was, "How can you leave <u>me</u> behind?"

Does she speak for all of my dear friends whom I'll soon hug goodbye? Could they really believe I'll allow our relationships to vanish?

Through the magic of airplane travel, e-mail, Facebook, and cell phones, our ties will endure. We are tightly bound; even the famous Houdini would fail to separate us.

THE GOLD LINE TO SOUTH PASADENA

"You'll have to forgive Grandma," I tell Felix. "I'll be calling you 'Is-Felix' for a few days."

My five-and-a-half-year old grandson flips his long hair from his eyes, pauses mid-bite, and waits for an explanation.

"You see, sweetheart, I've know Isaac for 18 years, so I'm used to that name. And even though he and I never lived in the same city, I saw him often enough to plant it in my head."

Felix takes another bite of his buttered French bread, and then patiently waits for more details.

We are sitting at an outdoor table in a bistro in South Pasadena. Jill -- his mother, my daughter -- is on her way back to our table and smiles as she sees up engaged in conversation. Her iPhone is pulled from her purse, and the image of small boy and grey-haired woman has quickly been saved and posted on Facebook.

The three of us have reached this destination after driving to a station in Chinatown, and then boarding the Gold Line to South Pasadena. Felix is enchanted by train rides and induces his mother to indulge him. I have been in town for just 24 hours, and although sleepy from pre-trip insomnia, do not forgo this chance to accompany them on the ride.

Jill places a Salad Nicoise on the table and leans in to hear the rest of my explanation for Felix's temporary tag. "So, until I get used to seeing you often, I'll probably start off by calling you by your brother's name. I'll catch myself and finish with your real name, and soon, you'll just be 'Felix.'"

My grandson appears to accept my excuse. His attention then turns to the trains passing by on a nearby track. Jill smiles; this makes sense to her, too. As for me, I am storing this scene on the plus side of evidence that I have made the right decision. Who could've imagined that two years after the death of my husband, Tommy, I would have moved from Chicago -- the city where I had lived nearly all of my 76 years -- to Los Angeles?

Although living walking distance to my daughter and her family was the primary reason for my move, I had a sense of something more propelling me forward, as if there was someone -- still unmet -- who needed my presence in L.A. I knew Jill and my grandsons were in solid shape and didn't require me, like some comic book heroine, to fly in and save the day.

But, perhaps there was a young woman, desperate for a faux Jewish mother, or someone stuck at a decision crossroad that involved me raising the gate?

That Gold Line ride was the penultimate event on my magical first Saturday morning in Los Angeles, which opened with a Torah study at a nearby Reform temple. This attempt to replicate my regular Chicago Shabbat experience turned out terrifically. A group of two-dozen men and women in my age group, some originally from my hometown, welcomed me.

Following that, I joined my grandson Isaac for a deli lunch at Grand Central Market in downtown L.A. This episode of sitting on a counter stool, eating a thick pastrami sandwich, with my tall, hip grandson at my right, filled me with a satiation that matched my appetite.

Sunday's schedule, two days post arrival, was similarly filled with happiness: a respite at Griffith Park while Jill hiked and I snacked and read the L.A. Times, then a visit to a pop-up restaurant with my son-in-law, Bruce, and my two grandsons.

A blank November calendar, which nagged with the possibility of boredom, is quickly becoming filled in. Along with Saturday mornings accounted for, I've had my first meeting for volunteers at Felix's school and will soon book a weekly tutoring date there.

Then, there's his birthday party on November 15, my book reading at Skylight Books on November 19, Thanksgiving at Jill's (my first ever in Los Angeles!), and tours of rental apartments in contention for my permanent residence.

As I think back on that first Saturday Gold Line train trip to South Pasadena, with my daughter and grandson seated a knee's length away, and all of the happenings of my first weekend in L.A., the identity of the person needing my presence here has become clear.

You've already guessed it, haven't you? It's me, of course.

PUBLIC TRANSIT

The patch on her right sleeve read "78866." Using the Pilot pen I had tucked into the notebook's spiral, I wrote down the number. "Let me repeat it," I said, "78866."

The conductor smiled as I continued, "I'm going to send a compliment to Metro. You've been terrific."

This was the second operator of a #2 Sunset-PCH bus that I had praised since my arrival in Los Angeles.

The first driver, per my request, called out my stop, even though the audio system alerted me several streets prior to reaching the corner of Hollywood and Poinsettia.

The episode with 78866 began when my Tap card was out of funds, but my Senior Citizen Pass could permit a 35-cent ride. "I don't have change," I told her, pulling a dollar bill from my wallet. (The day before, my grandson, Felix, had showed me his treasure chest of coins, so I emptied my change purse into it.) "Just take the dollar; my fault for being unprepared," I told her.

"Just ask one of the passengers for change," she said. "Don't waste money."

"No, that's fine. My mistake."

But, 78866 insisted; so curbing embarrassment, I called out my request, which was quickly answered by a mother cuddling her baby.

She nimbly used her free hand to extract coins, at first refusing my paper bill, but accepting after I pressed it into her palm.

Of course, there have been hiccups on my use of Metro. On Sunday, after alighting from the #704 at Santa Monica and Fairfax, I asked a friendly woman where I would catch the #218. It wasn't until my 35-cents had plunked that I had learned I would've been travelling in the opposite direction of my destination in Studio City.

I relate these experiences because prior to moving to Los Angeles, various people warned me against its public transit system. "Dicey passengers, unreliable service," they cautioned. "You'll need to buy a car."

However, I had received my Carless Basic Training in Chicago and was determined to avoid the expense. Uber had successfully been my option for short trips, but for longer excursions, I turned to Metro.

My initial reasons to go carless in L.A. included: a desire to save money, to get exercise walking to bus stops and coffee shops, to learn its landscape via window seats, and to prove my independence. But I now realize it was my childhood adventures that bonded me to public transit.

It started in the 1940's, with the red Pullman streetcar that stopped on tracks outside our mom-and-pop grocery store. Here are excerpts, via my memoir, that may help you understand our relationship:

"Once on board the streetcar, Mother took a quarter from her purse and handed it to the conductor who made change for the ten-cent fare with the coin holder he wore on his belt.

"Then, with the car in motion, we lurched through the aisle until we found two empty spaces. After we landed on the cane-backed seats, I tugged at Mother's coat sleeve and said, 'Look, there's Mrs. Schwartz, she's going into the A&P.'"

Okay, that particular passage is a bit dour because it previewed the coming demise of our small establishment that couldn't compete with supermarkets. But there are other paragraphs that can enlighten.

Here's one from Chapter 7 of "The Division Street Princess":

"I recalled the first time Estherly and I rode the streetcar, on our own, to Wabash Avenue downtown for dance lessons.

"Dressed in outfits a step up from school clothes and carrying our tap shoes in drawstring sacks, we thought we were big shots.

"My cousin and I had a shtick back then that we adlibbed every time the streetcar approached the bridge over the Chicago River.

"'It's going up,' Estherly would cry out, as the trolley paused at the water's edge. While we'd watch the jaws of the bridge unfold and reach for the sky, and the tall sails slip below the open bridge, Estherly would add, 'What if it doesn't shut back down tight? What if it falls apart when we cross it, and we plunge into the river?'

"'I can't swim,' I would wail, and clutch Estherly's sleeve as if I were a starlet in a B movie. 'Save me!' Once the streetcar made it safely over the closed bridge, we'd laugh at our pretend terror.

So, to all those who warned me against Los Angeles' Metro, you should know that once the red Pullman, streetcar tracks, and overhead cables, have been imprinted on your childhood brain, it's useless dissuading the rider from the joys of staring out the window, watching her world -- old and new -- pass before her enchanted eyes.

TREASURE HUNT

My favorite clue was "kitty in a tree." I think Felix liked that one, too, because he asked that the Hello Kitty key fob be used in three more games.

It all started with a text from Jill: "Can you come over and hang out with Felix for awhile?" The previous day, she had hosted a large Thanksgiving dinner, and was hoping to catch up on needed rest. "I'll try and get a babysitter, but are you available until then?"

Her query arrived while I was riding a bus that would get me to a hardware store.

I was seeking a garage door opener that my daughter could use to park in the space allotted to my new apartment. Happy visions of her dropping over spontaneously were spurred by long ago memories of the times in Chicago when I'd return home to find either of my daughters' cars parked outside.

On the bus, I was studying directions to the store and was as focused as if I were a gold rush prospector. But after receiving Jill's request, I shifted to my attention to my iPhone and typed: "Happy to help. On way to Baller's on Hyperion. Will text when done. Pick me up there."

This new plan heartened me, because four weeks into my move to Los Angeles, I was intent on being an asset, rather than a burden. If I could be helpful -- by entertaining my grandson and providing a respite to my daughter -- my immigration could be considered a win-win.

When I completed my purchases, that included a dry mop and a just-in-case toilet plunger, I typed: "Ready to be retrieved."

"Isaac's on his way." This alert from my daughter was another perk -- a chance to see my 18-year-old grandson whose words, "Why don't you move to L.A.?" sparked my recent long-distance transfer.

"Can you get Felix off his screen?" were Jill's first words after her welcoming hug. I followed her gaze to my six-year-old grandson who was prone on the couch, his eyes focused on an electronic pad and his thumbs swiftly pressing buttons.

I put my hands on my hips and surveyed the indoor scene. I considered my daughter's challenge as one crucial for me to accept and win. But first, I had to lure Felix outside.

While he continued his game, I took a few moments to contemplate their backyard. It held a lemon tree, Ping-Pong table, hammock, outdoor sofa, potted plants, a coiled water hose, and other items I could foresee as props in a game.

"How about a treasure hunt?" I said to Felix. He lifted his head to face me -- interested, but not yet ready to abandon his screen. "I'll hide things, then I'll draw a map with clues. You'll have to search to find them. If you collect all, you'll win a prize."

To be honest, I had never devised, played, or completed such a game. Also, I can only draw stick figures and animals that can be identified by humps, feathers, or wings. But, I was undaunted.

Felix must've assumed I was a whiz at this sort of sport, for he quickly rolled off the couch to round up paper and markers. "You stay inside and close your eyes," I said, as I walked around the living room scouting potential treasures.

Along with the kitty key fob, in a jumble of small toys, I found a plastic boat, a cotton stalk of celery, and a mini motorcycle with one wheel missing.

I quickly placed the kitty in the crook of the tree, the boat near the water hose, the motorcycle along the Ping-Pong net, and in what I considered a flash of inspiration, tucked the celery behind Isaac who was lounging on the hammock.

Then, I sketched out the map, and listed clues. Along with "kitty in a tree," I wrote, "boat needs water," "cycle gets a paddle," and "celery loves a boy."

"Come out now," I shouted to Felix. He ran from the house and grabbed the map, which looked to me as if one of his kindergarten pals had drawn it. As he raced through the yard, I'd shout an occasional, "you're warm" or a more helpful "turn around."

When he had successfully gathered all of the hidden toys, he raised his hands in triumph, and then continued for three more rounds with new objects and clues.

From the corner of my eye, I could see Jill watching us. Her face bore an expression reminiscent of the one I had when I had spotted her Honda outside my home all those years ago. It appears we all struck gold.

COIN-OPERATED LAUNDRY

I opened the lid of the Maytag Commercial, measured half a capful of Tide with Downy, and dumped into the machine, my shopping cart full of bathroom towels and rugs. Then, I pulled six quarters out of my change purse and slid each into the slot. When I heard the tub fill with water, I felt as proud as if I had just been handed my college degree.

"This is a scene I never expected to witness," said Tommy. I had conjured my deceased spouse for this episode because I knew he would enjoy the sight of his Jewish Princess in a coin-operated laundry.

My mother, a neighbor of his in heaven -- who evidently couldn't resist an opportunity to jibe -- weighed in. "Somehow I thought your relocation to Los Angeles would move you up a notch," she said. The tone was familiar, one I recognized from my childhood that usually accompanied, "Stand up straight," or "Comb you hair."

"Why have you two teamed up to rain on my parade?" I said. "Couldn't you let my pride sustain for at least one cycle? I'm pleased I'm not thrown by this lowly chore after enjoying in-home laundry for the past three decades."

"You're right," Tommy said, "but I remember how sorry you felt for me when I told you I once spent every Friday night at the Laundromat.

"I can still see your tender expression after I moved into your townhouse and you escorted me to your washer and dryer."

I hit pause on this dearly departed dialogue to recall the setting he described. It was 1996 and we had enjoyed a whirlwind romance. Tommy, only a few weeks after our first date, transferred clothes and favorite furniture from the apartment he lived in down the block to my place. We were both singles in our 60's -- he a long-time divorcé, me recently separated after a 30-year marriage -- and our compatibility encouraged a leap.

Although we were compatible, and did have similar opinions in music, television, plays, and pets; Tommy and I differed in religion and income.

It was the last mismatch that I intended to remedy. I would groom my second husband to be a Jewish prince. There would be no more Friday nights sitting in a chair at the Laundromat with his latest paperback mystery as companion. With me, came a willing laundress who was tickled to offer this perk to my sweetie.

Along with the in-home washer and dryer, I pressured my prince to accept a new suit for our wedding, a set of golf clubs to replace his vintage batch, and his own Honda Accord.

I mention these, not to extol my generosity, but to emphasize that Tommy didn't request these gifts, didn't care about money, and would've married me with none of my perks. But, I was so delighted to be with such a low-maintenance guy, whose only goal was to make me happy, that it brought me pleasure to shower him.

"Such a sweet story," my mother said, yawning at my exposition. "I like Tommy, don't get me wrong," she said, winking at him. "But I had hoped that for your second marriage, you would've landed someone who would spend money on *you*. You can't blame me for that."

Then, she wrapped an arm around her son-in-law, and fixed a red-stained kiss on his cheek. Tommy, who appreciated attractive women -- and Mother was a knockout -- smirked.

"And now, we find you in a dreary laundry room off of the garage, feeding quarters into machines. This is not where I expected to find you," she said.

"Just like you didn't count on a life behind the counter of a mom-and-pop grocery store," I said. Mother's face changed. I had erred in reminding her of those years when she struggled to keep our business afloat while my happy-to-lucky dad steered it into one debt-laden boulder after another.

"Sorry, Mom," I said. "I know you just want the best for me. But, despite this laundry room, I'm really enjoying my Los Angeles apartment and life.

"I get to see more of your granddaughters and great-grandchildren, and I don't have to deal with Chicago's winter."

This brightened her; Tommy was smiling, too. Now it was my turn to grin as he took his mother-in-law's hand and said, “Okay, Min, time to go back. So, she’s down here doing her laundry. If she can live with that, we shouldn’t complain.” Then he added, “Love you, sweetheart,” and faded from my imagination.

“Me, too,” Mom said, and before she disappeared, gave my cheek the red twin of Tommy’s.

HAPPY HOLIDAYS

I was the seventh resident to tape a greeting card to the wall of our building's elevator. The design I had selected, and affixed with double-sided Scotch tape, was as holiday-neutral as the others: Snowman, Santa, a sprig of holly (mine), and wintry scenes. No figure on the cross, crèche, or menorah.

When I first saw the cards on the elevator wall, which bore people's first names only and their apartment number, I thought, *how quaint.* At the time, it didn't occur to me to join in on the display because I had only been a resident for a few weeks.

Although I had introduced myself to several neighbors on my walkway, and said hello to fellow passengers in this small elevator, I didn't feel long-term enough to post a greeting card. (I feel a need to explain the use of "walkway" rather than "floor," which would've been the terminology in a high-rise. But I live in a 24-unit building, which is square-shaped and overlooks a ground floor landscaped courtyard. To me, it's very film noire.)

But on this elevator day, after going up-and-down several times to do my laundry, I decided, *why not?* My card read, "Happy Holidays." I added in pen, "to all!" and signed Elaine, #21.

Some background: I have lived and adjusted, in a variety of neighborhoods; I count 15 since 1960, the year of my first marriage. This condominium building, which houses a few other renters like myself, is my latest challenge. I have a one-year lease -- enough time to plant myself and see if I flourish. Or, if I'm seasonal, like the holly on my card.

One nourishment -- along with my family -- is the fact that I have settled in a fertile neighborhood called "Beachwood." My daughters and her friends have told me that this is the place where they all docked when they first moved as a troupe from Chicago to L.A.

I like the idea that I'm in a setting of fresh starts, hopefulness, and even youthful enthusiasm, even though I've topped all newcomers' ages by several decades. Why can't this also be blossoming soil for the older set?

In an earlier essay, I claimed I wanted to find a place that was walking distance from my daughter Jill. I thought the proximity would ensure an easy transition from my former home and life in Chicago, and that I could untangle any familial knots and knit a new tapestry of family love so tight, it'd be impossible to unravel.

So, while I was temporarily housed in an Airbnb that *was* walking distance from my kin in Silver Lake, I reviewed half a dozen places nearby. Alas, none felt like *home.*

But, as soon as I stepped into this Beachwood apartment, I sent a text to Jill: "it's perfect." When she -- in a reversal of roles that had her playing the scrutinizing mother and me the silent daughter -- came for a viewing, she agreed and the year's lease was signed.

So, instead of walking distance to Jill, I'm a 30-minute bus ride (#2 along Sunset Blvd.) or a 10-minute Uber or Lyft car ride ($8) to her home. But in the swap of neighborhoods, while losing easy access to dear relatives, I gained a grocery store a block away (the amazing Gelson's), a comedy club, (Upright Citizens Brigade), and a second-hand bookstore (Counterpoint where I bought Alice Munro's "Friend of My Youth").

Another bonus of my new home -- that helps to make up for the distance from Jill -- is that I'm a 15-minute walk from buses that can take me to several favorites: Temple Israel of Hollywood, a reform synagogue for Saturday morning Torah study, to Target on La Brea, or to The Grove on 3rd and Fairfax with its Farmers Market and Apple store.

And recently, I walked 1.3 miles to The Trails coffee shop in lush Griffith Park. It's that benefit that has me grateful for my locale, for from opposite directions, mother and daughter recently met for coffee, conversation, and hugs.

Eventually, the holiday cards that are decorating the elevator will be tugged down. Perhaps before that happens, passengers will take a moment to flip the cover of each card and read the name of the signer. Most will have no clue about "Elaine." I figure I have the coming new year to correct that mystery; not only for my neighbors, but also for resident 21 herself.

THE CREW ON YUCCA STREET

If I hadn't seen his foot peeking out from the heap, I wouldn't have known there was a man asleep under the jumble of blankets.

And, if I hadn't ventured into the roadway to call back a tiny dog that was sniffing Yucca Street and dodging cars, I wouldn't have heard a woman's squawk rise from another mountain of covers near the first spot.

After I had coaxed the dog out of the road, I heard her say. "Come back here." It wasn't a shout, because she had likely just been woken by my unfamiliar voice. Her own speech still has curtains of sleep blurring the words.

After the dog returned to its owner and concocted shelter, I continued my walk, which was taking me from my Los Angeles apartment to Hollywood and Vine. Along with the dog and the pair under blankets, the sights on my route included the Capitol tower, which is shaped like a stack of records on a turntable and commemorates its artists, including Nate King Cole, Billie Holiday, and Ella Fitzgerald. The Yucca crew can also easily see the building from their jerry-rigged vantage point.

I am carless in my new city -- a decision based on funds, and a hunger for exercise and exploration - and take this road nearly every day.

While I'm pleased how my move to the West Coast is turning out, scenes like the one on Yucca and similar encampments on nearly every corner, on bus stop benches, and under every freeway overpass and onramps, are dimming its gloss.

"What's with all of the homeless in L.A.?" I asked family and friends. Shrugs and raised hands of helplessness met my query. "Maybe it's because you all drive so you don't see them," I added. "But with my walking and bus rides, they seem to be everywhere."

In my former life in Chicago, where I lived in a downtown neighborhood, I had encountered panhandlers with outstretched coffee cups or hand-written appeals. At one point, I prepped for these strolls with a pocket of dollar bills. When my $5 cache emptied, I'd have to turn a blind eye to pleas. That was about it for my aid.

The Los Angeles tableaus are different. They range from one ragged person propped against a storefront, to clusters of people and shopping carts piled with empty bottles, cans, mattresses, clothing, and stuff likely culled from dumpsters.

The question of how this came to be in such a rich and scenic city wouldn't evaporate in my brain, so I decided to investigate. If I could learn more about the downfalls that left people living on the street, and programs underway to address the issue, maybe I could find a way to be part of the solution.

Here are some things I've learned so far:

+The Los Angeles Homeless Services Authority, a city-county agency, oversees $70 million in state, local and national funding for housing and other services.

+The federal homeless funding formula penalizes Los Angeles by factoring in the age of the housing stock. For example, Philadelphia gets $11,000 per homeless person, while Los Angeles get $1,500.

+On any given night in LA County, there are 58,000 homeless, of which 3,000 -- 4,000 are over the age of 62, with 33% of them women. (Could that ever happen to my friends? To me?)

+L.A. has the country's largest homeless veteran population -- 2,600 -- and Mayor Eric Garcetti has promised to house them by the end of 2015.

+Social Security payments and low wage jobs are barely enough to find permanent housing. Many landlords of subsidized units are reluctant to rent to those who are homeless.

+The absence of a permanent address makes it extremely difficult to get a job.

And, here are some steps I'm taking:

> +I've volunteered on January 29 to assist in the 2015 Greater Los Angeles Point-In-Time Homeless Count. This project helps determine how many people nightly sleep on the street.
>
> +I plan to try and meet staff of organizations that intrigue me, including Shelter Partnership, Homeless Health Care Los Angeles, and the Skid Row Housing Trust. This variety should broaden my knowledge.

In a few months after my research, maybe I'll introduce myself to the Yucca crew. If I learn their names, and that of their dog, I can call him back if he wanders into the street again. Maybe hearing his name will pull him quicker away from danger.

THIS ROOMMATE FEELS FAMILIAR

Her red Van canvas shoes, size 7, are parked under the chair in the hallway. They are nestled next to my weathered Sacony running shoes, size 5. Every morning, when I wake in my Los Angeles apartment, and spy our shoes side-by-side, I feel happy. It's the sensation that originated decades ago when I recovered from anesthesia and was informed, *it's a girl.*

My daughter, Faith, was my firstborn, into the world 18 months before her sister, Jill. For half of the year, Faith lives in Boston, with her 12-year-old daughter, Betsy, and their extended family. This is Faith's second season writing on her sister Jill's Amazon Series, "Transparent." Instead of couch surfing like she did during Season One, she has accepted my invitation to be my roommate.

"We'll see how it goes," I had said, when upon arriving in L.A., I opted to seek a larger apartment that could accommodate the two of us, rather than a studio for just me. I was pretty confident the arrangement would work -- Faith is an easygoing sort of gal -- and that the money she would contribute to my rent would make the tab easier for me.

"I'm sure it'll be fine, Momma," she said. I should mention she is also sweetly optimistic.

I insisted Faith take the one bedroom for herself because I wake at 4 a.m. and jump into my home office. I purchased an IKEA sofa bed, which is providing me with excellent sleep. "It's my own studio," I say, when she repeats her guilt for taking the bedroom.

"I can get up, turn on lights, make coffee, write in my journal, and get on my laptop. I couldn't do that if you were on the sofa bed," I add, smug about my longtime routine.

Of course, we've each had to make compromises to oblige our lifestyles. I watch my critically acclaimed TV shows before she gets home from work.

Then, I turn the remote over to her for reality shows. "The Celebrity Apprentice," "The Real Housewives of Atlanta" and "Beverly Hills" are her favorites.

Faith turns off the living room television at 8 p.m. when it's lights out for this early bird. Often, I'll lounge on the opened sofa bed and try to watch her shows, but having Donald Trump being the last image you see before dreamland is not something I'd recommend.

I don't insist that Faith make her bed or tidy up her room before she leaves for work. It's a method I employed when she and her sister were toddlers: I just close the door. I suppose I should tell you I was a calm parent, madly in love with my two daughters. In my eyes, they could do no wrong.

I raised them without judgment because I wanted to do the opposite of my mother. Their grandmother undoubtedly loved me, but her criticism of my weight, my slouch, and other attributes that reminded her of my father, who she nagged often, wounded me.

I was also guided by a classic parenting book, "Children The Challenge," by Rudolf Dreikurs. His lessons "natural consequences" and "let the children handle their own battles" suited my style. Consequently, I never interfered if they were fussing with each other. I simply stayed out of their disagreements, and encouraged them to figure out how to reach a satisfactory conclusion.

Back to the adjustments as a roommate: Faith has to remind me, "Please close the bathroom door, Momma."

I reply, "Oh, sorry, I'm so used to living on my own." But, this is false, for when Tommy was alive, we never closed the bathroom door. In fact, I think that was one of my favorite parts about our compatible 14-year-marriage. Keep the bathroom door open to continue conversations. For comfort, dispense of my bra when in the house. Leave on the hall table the baseball cap that covered his balding dome.

Actually, in many ways Faith reminds me of the pleasure and ease of living with Tommy. There's the heart bounce when the front door opens and a familiar voice announces, "I'm home", and their appreciation of my simple dinners. Tommy would gladly eat anything I cooked; my daughter is grateful for the Gelson's-prepared food that awaits her at day's end.

These comparisons bring up another reminder: Tommy's size 9 running shoes would sit at the bottom of the stairs in our Chicago house. That's where I would perch, too, to remove my 5's. Two pair of shoes nestled side-by-side; what could be sweeter, or so familiar.

THE HAT

The hat cost $35, more than I had hoped to spend. But this straw Fedora that I found at a stall at The Grove had the advantage of an adjustable interior band, which could be pulled tighter, making it smaller. This feature -- devised by the Chinese manufacturer -- created a hat that would fit my teensy head.

So, I sprung for it. I had been seeking such a hat for weeks. I was worried that my constant baseball cap wearing was thinning my hair.

Although a Google search denied baseball caps as the culprits, the fact that I had been wearing them daily against Los Angeles' strong sun, pointed to those canvas covers as guilty parties.

"We all lose some hair as we get older," my daughter, Faith, who has a luscious head of dark brown hair, said.

"But, you can't see it on your head," I said. "With my gray hair, my scalp shows all of the empty places."

I figured that the straw hat, with a weave that allows air to flow through, would not create the heat generated by a baseball cap. Perhaps, my disappearing shoots would magically reappear.

So although the Fedora was purchased as sort of a prescription, I soon found that it was bringing me other benefits: people were stopping me on the street, or calling out from cars with, "Hey, I like your hat!"

With each salute, I'd preen like a beauty queen, which reminded me of my husband Tommy and his Stetson. I can't remember where we bought it, but it's easy for me to recall my late husband's adoration of that hat. Normally, he was a baseball cap kind of guy, and we had upper closet shelves full of imprinted varieties to confirm that. There were dozens hawking colleges, towns, golf courses, and museums.

When we met in 1996, Tommy was already losing his hair. He often told this silly joke: *I have wavy hair; it's waving me goodbye.* Those in earshot would groan, but that didn't stop him from repeating it whenever he got the chance. And because I found him to be so compatible, so endearing, I'd grin, no matter the number of reruns.

After we married in 1998, and he continued to lose his hair, I urged him to shave it all off. "It's sexy," I would say. What I kept to myself was, *Please stop with the comb overs.*

Tommy saved his beloved Stetson for evenings out and he would pair it with a leather jacket. This combo pleased him so much, that whenever he'd don this outfit, he'd spend a few minutes sashaying in front of the open hall closet doors.

After Tommy died, and before I left the house we lived in together, I had an estate sale. "Estate" is really a misnomer. The home we shared was a modest three-bedroom, two-story, with a large back yard and front porch. I'm not sure why you need to know that; it's just that I like to resurrect that image whenever I find an opening.

Anyway, now that I've made both of us sad with that picture of lost domesticity, here's another teary tidbit: I included all of my husband's clothing in that sale, including his Stetson. I don't know why I did that; why couldn't I have held on to the Stetson? I have his ashes, his watch, his wedding ring, and his wallet. I could've added the Stetson to the mini-memorial I've set up on my nightstand. But, you're right; maybe it would've been too much.

When I leave the house now, and place my Fedora upon my evidently smaller than normal head, I don't do the cute dance Tommy used to do. But, I do admit to a bit of showing off in front of the round mirror in my entry hall. I have to do some adjusting before my exit, for although the hat fits width-wise, it is somewhat tall, so I squish it down a bit to look just so.

Of course I wish I could have Tommy on my arm with his Stetson. We'd be an adorable pair; each hat covering up our steady hair loss. But, that's not to be, so I'll wear my straw and tip it to my guy who taught me how to stylishly wear a hat.

GAME

The only sounds I could hear were the clacking of small Bakelite tiles and the calls of "crack, bam, dot" from the four women seated around the table. As I peeked over the shoulder of one of the players, who was allowing this learner to sit in, I studied the designs on the vivid squares filling the center of the table.

The tiles were imprinted with Chinese characters and symbols, and the women's exclamations came as each one discarded a tile she had picked up, or one plucked from the rack facing her.

You may recognize that I was observing the ancient game of Mah Jongg. What you may not fathom is what Elaine Soloway was doing at the table. For wasn't she the gal who swore she shunned card-, table-, and hide and seek- games? Isn't this the former Chicagoan who insisted she hadn't the patience for anything lasting longer than 30 minutes?

Moreover, isn't she the Los Angeles transplant who declared she preferred solitary, rather than group pursuits, especially those not under her control?

So what are we to make of this picture of our Elaine perched on the edge at several Mah Jongg games, her view focused on her teacher's line-up and folder outlining the possible hands.

Sit for a bit, as I pull back the curtain to this recent phenomenon when I (time to switch to first person) decided to discard all of my restrictions, including my previous snobbery about the game.

My conversion -- aptly enough -- came at a weekend retreat for the women of Temple Israel of Hollywood. That's the synagogue I attend for Saturday morning Torah study.

My friend Thelma, who chauffeurs me for the weekly lessons, urged me to sign up for the retreat. "You'll get a chance to meet women of all ages and enjoy the Ojai scenery and clean air," she said.

I hesitated before agreeing, because as I have stated, I was a non-joiner; and on top of that, was not a camper. Although there were opportunities to attend summer sleepover camp during my childhood, I was a scaredy-cat. I never wanted to leave my mama; and since I was slightly pudgy and uncoordinated, I preferred for my school vacations the concrete sidewalks of Division Street or the greenery of Humboldt Park.

Despite all that, something spurred me to sign up for the weekend retreat, which offered exercise classes, Jewish learning, hikes, and Mah Jongg. But the first entry in my journal on the morning after check-in, read: *I have made a mistake. I don't belong here. Everyone knows more about Judaism than I. Where will I get my coffee when I wake before breakfast? I can't figure out the heat in this room. I wish I could leave early.*

Oy, such a complainer! Even I got tired of me. Then, I said to myself: *Would it kill you to get with the program? Go to beginner Mah Jongg! Instead of whining, be game.*

So, I did, and as I sat at the table with women decades younger than myself, I imagined my dearly departed mother and her sisters hovering overhead. I could almost hear Min, Rose, Etta, and Molly clicking the tiles. I could listen to their conversations, gossip, and laughter. I could practically smell their perfume. I easily saw their beautiful faces -- pinup girls all of them -- and their smiles as they relished their time together.

Let's pause for a bit of history: While Mah Jongg originated in China in the 19th century; it became part of Jewish life during World War II. In fact, 12 Jewish women who raised money at tournaments for various relief organizations formed the National Mah Jongg League. The game spread in the 1950s and 1960s to our mothers' card tables. And currently, it's popular among younger women. For example, my Ojai teachers were in their '30's and '40's.

Now, I'm not sure if I'll ever really learn the game or even play it again. But, that's not the moral of this story. It is this: sometimes you can leave your comfort zone and try something you've previously avoided. Sometimes, you can say to yourself: *would it hurt you to play? Would it be a disaster to stay awake past your normal bedtime? Could you possibly enjoy being part of a group? Would it kill you to take directions from someone other than yourself?*

As for my misgivings cited in my Day One journal, it turned out that I loved the Shabbat services, despite not knowing the Hebrew lyrics and melodies, I joined new friends at an early morning coffee run, and the low heat setting in my room kept me toasty.

Crack, bam, dot!

WOOF

A 33-lb. bag of Science Diet costs $48 at the Petco on Hollywood and Bronson. I could skip that store and instead purchase a natural product recommended by the salesperson at Tailwaggers on Franklin, but that food might be more expensive.

I don't own a dog, but lately I've been haunting pet stores and imagining that I indeed have one. Not a large breed like Sasha or Buddy, the Golden Retrievers that once lived with Tommy and me, but instead, a mid-sized Rescue. (Our dogs died at ages 9 and 14, their male owner at 77.)

Currently, I am renting a condo in Los Angeles, and my lease states that pets aren't allowed, so my store visits are more like fantasies. But, I have declared that at lease end, I will move to an apartment that permits dogs.

Having said that, I will foster a dog.

By visiting the Adoption Fairs on occasional Saturdays at Tailwaggers, I've learned that an organization -- Dogs Without Borders -- "will supply all food, flea meds, leashes, collars, tags, and any vet needs throughout the fostering process. If you are fostering puppies, you will also be supplied with crates/pens and puppy pads. Food and care items are typically delivered with the dog and you are then resupplied at Adoption Fairs."

Doesn't that make you feel better? It did me; it reduces my skittishness at the cost of the 33-lb. bag of Science Diet and doodads that I was ogling. Also, I won't pick a puppy; it's an older dog for me. Tommy and I adopted Buddy at age 1-1/2. He was already housebroken, and I think because he was labeled an adult when we welcomed into our loving embraces, he was the sweetest, easiest dog ever.

Sasha, who was a purebred, was a bit of a handful from puppy to senior. We loved her dearly, but she did not like other dogs. And if you have such a temperamental bitch (allowed language), you know how difficult is to walk that sassy girl without her threatening to harass or bite another pooch. But, I must credit Sasha for leading me to Tommy. You see; he and I lived on the same street. It was 1996, I was divorced from my first spouse, and I was an early morning dog walker. Tommy was a fitness buff and jogged at the same hour. So every time we'd meet in the purple darkness, he would stop and pet Sasha. One thing led to another, and you know the rest of the story.

"Why do you want a dog?" my daughter, Jill, had asked when I was first pitching the idea. "You can come over and cuddle ours whenever you need a fix."

Jill's two giant Labradoodles are indeed lovable, but I'm seeking a mid-sized dog to hang out at my house; one who will welcome me with ecstatic whoops when I enter, and who will jump onto my bed at nighttime. (In my mind, there is no reason to have a dog if he/she can't be on the bed; same with furniture. But, that's just me.)

My other daughter, Faith, said, "Do you really want the hassle? Whenever you're out, you'll have to rush home to walk the dog. Do you need that?"

I know my kids are trying to get me to slow down and think rationally -- actions completely foreign to my personality. What they don't understand is: despite my moving to Los Angeles to be closer to this family, these dear ones cannot assuage my particular loneliness.

Oh, I can book lunches with new friends every day of the week and I can visit with my concerned kin any time I desire. And, I can hug my grandchildren at will. But if you've experienced the emptiness once filled by a loving husband and a loyal, funny dog, you understand the void.

As any dog owner will tell you, potential spouses aren't the only humans one can attract with a canine at the end of your leash. Friends! At nearly every neighborhood I've lived in, there was at least one new furry friend for dog, and one charming person for me. Perhaps we'll meet our duo at my next apartment building?

The only problem I can envision with my plan is the possibility of falling in love with my foster pet. What happens then to my budget? The $48 bags of Science Diet? The meds, leash, treats, vets bills that won't be funded if pooch and I skip from foster to adoption? Well, how about all of us just sitting and staying for now? Good girl. Good boy.

SLEEPING AROUND

One queen-sized bed, one foldout couch, one double-sized bed, one futon, and one king-sized bed. These are places where I rested my head on a recent visit to hometown Chicago. My initial motivation in accepting invitations from five dear ones was to save hotel fees. And, while it might have been easier to settle into just one of the proffered rooms, and not have to schlep luggage from car trunk to car trunk, each visit brought its own reward: a chance to deeply bond with my host. For despite being acquainted with these friends for years -- that ranged from three to sixty-five -- we rarely had the luxury that dozens of uninterrupted hours could bring.

Each morning, as I drank coffee that was thoughtfully prepared the night before, I'd listen for the opening of a bedroom door, the sound of slippered feet coming my way, and the familiar greeting from a bathrobed friend.

As I'd watch each enter her kitchen, pull a mug from a cabinet, and pour her hot drink, I felt as if I had been reunited with a long-lost sister. But it wasn't DNA that matched us, simply years of traveling together through life's joys and sorrows. A trio of these friends had known me through first marriage and divorce, and all cleaved to me through my second husband's illness and death.

In the dark Evanston, Morton Grove, and Chicago mornings, we'd bring each other up-to-date on the goings on during the nearly five months since I departed from my longtime home. And even though I chat frequently with these friends, and view Facebook status reports, these early morning kitchen conversations were as precious as an heirloom.

These recent scenes were what I had been attempting to create many years ago with my daughters. When I was still living in Chicago and they would visit from Boston or Los Angeles, I would plead for them to stay at our house. After all, Tommy and I had a spare room with a queen--sized bed that was decorated with photographs and paintings of these girls and their families. I would often joke to my friends that this space was a shrine to my kids.

I tried to explain the joy of seeing a loved room slowly drift down the stairs from the second floor to the kitchen, where I had been up for hours. Their hair tossed like brunette haystacks, eyes still sleepy from travel and time differences, crinkly tee shirts and shorts serving as pajamas, and faces still unfolded from sleep.

While one daughter easily accepted my invitation, the other insisted on a hotel. "I'll be over first thing in the morning," she'd promise.

"It's not the same thing," I'd say into the phone, my left hand cradling cheek and chin. How could I explain that the showered, dressed, and put-together young woman who would be ringing my doorbell was not the one I had longed to envelop?

Once though, when both daughters were traveling with their children, the recalcitrant gal agreed to stay over. I can still see my grandchildren leaping from bed to air mattress, jumps that doubled my delight.

After Tommy died and I moved to my River North high rise, one of its bonuses was a fully furnished guest apartment. I was in heaven! Now, just 10 floors down from my 19th floor unit, my clan was tucked in for easy access. As soon as I'd wake, I'd check my cell phone to learn who was up, who wanted coffee, and who was available for breakfast. Although they weren't within my four walls, I could win the early morning scenes I relished.

Now that I live in Los Angeles and are about three miles away from my offspring, I will frequently hire a Lyft or Uber to take me in the 6 a.m. darkness to their house. Along with my just-awoken daughters, I now am blessed with grandchildren still wearing their own nighttime outfits, their hair adorably messed, and yawns intermixed with "Hi, Grandma."

In a few months, I'll likely venture from LA and return to Chicago to again see my left-behind dear friends. Because I was a good guest -- stripped linens and picked up an occasional restaurant check -- I assume their queen-, double, foldout, futon, and king-sized beds will welcome me. If not, could I sleep at your place? An air mattress will do, but you must promise a first-in-the-morning cup of coffee with a sisterly hug for me.

YMCA: THEN, NOW

I used a fingernail to lift the silver circle on the key ring. When there was enough of an opening, I pushed the hole in my new YMCA fob through the circle until it closed and sealed.

That's when I felt a tap on my shoulder, soft as a feather, but familiar.

"Finally." It was the voice of Tommy making himself heard in my head at the Hollywood-Wilshire YMCA.

My response to my deceased husband was mental, rather than aloud, as I didn't want those in earshot to think me loony. "I knew you'd show up at the Y," I said, as I pictured Tommy in his tank top and shorts, his body trim with muscled biceps and calves.

At once, the small chest of drawers that stood at his side of our bed appeared in my mind's eye; second drawer; that's where his gym clothes lived. Neat piles of tank tops and shorts, most purchased from thrift shops, for my husband of 14 years was as slim in his spending as he was in body.

I could see him choosing the outfit he appeared in during this imaginary visit. First, he'd have removed from the closet the gym bag he had used during his 40-year membership at Chicago's Lakeview Y. His weathered shoes would already be stowed, along with a towel. Would he find the note I had left him?

Tommy taught me that. At the beginning of our romance -- both in our 60's at the time -- he would write tender Post-its and hide them for me to find sometime during my day. Imagine, at that mature age, being reminded there was this fellow who thought I walked on water.

I hadn't learned this sentimentality previously, but I leaped in, stowing my own notes to Tommy in one of his gym shoes, or in a drawer, surprises I knew would light his morning.

Sadly, it's not all mushy stuff when I recall my guy and his beloved Y in Chicago. Much of that switched to spy games after he was diagnosed with Frontotemporal Degeneration and lost his ability to speak.

To be certain I would be contacted if anything happened to him when he was not under my watch, I bought him a medical ID bracelet. The band's metal plate was engraved with his name, his illness, and my cell phone number.

But, my Tommy refused to wear the band. I didn't pressure him because I figured the gym was his sanctuary, free of a hovering wife. It was the place where he didn't have to talk; where he was proud of his three times a week attendance, and routine of 33 minutes on the elliptical, then 20 minutes of weight lifting. At the Y, he was a strongman, not someone needing a medical ID bracelet.

"Hel-lo, are you still here?" It was my fictional Tommy waking me from a scene that he evidently didn't want to revisit.

"Sorry, honey," I said, miffed at myself for clouding his drop in. "Were you surprised to see me here, signing up at a Y rather than some fancy health club?"

"I knew you'd come around eventually," he said. "Sure L.A.'s sunshine is great and the glitter is fun, but I knew you'd wind up in a place that felt comfortable, familiar. And affordable."

Ah yes, there was my budget-minded buddy reminding me of my, um, tendency to fudge finances. "Have you been keeping an eye on me since I landed in California? Were you worried I'd be living on credit cards and wishful thinking?"

"Well, I can't say it hadn't entered my mind," he said. "But, it's more than the low membership fee that makes me happy to see you here. It reminds me of the days we'd go to the Y together. Remember when we first married, the time I took you on a tour and showed you how to operate each machine?"

"Of course I remember," I said, as the slideshow slipped across my vision. Before then, Tommy had been a long-time bachelor, and I felt his pride as he paused in his instructions to introduce me to all of his gym pals.

"My wife," he'd say, puffed as if he had won the state's lotto.

"He's the best," his cronies would say.

In real time, my Strength Class was about to begin, so I shook my head to tuck my spouse back to my brain.

I entered the Women's Locker Room and placed my belongings in an empty space. But before closing the lock, I rummaged through my gym bag to be certain I hadn't left anything behind. My fingers probed each corner.

Could a long-ago note be hiding somewhere? Nope, all gone.

HOW TO FIGHT

I hung up on her. Our 30-minute battle exhausted me and I needed to retreat. Instead of a neutral corner, where a trainer urging me to re-enter the ring would tend to me, I dropped into the cushion of my lounge chair. My abrupt halt to our cell phone conversation didn't make me feel like a champ; instead, I felt flattened, as if I were an over-the-hill boxer.

I returned to the paused TV show I had been watching before the phone call.

As the images on the screen moved from scene to scene, and characters' voices bounced from one to another, I realized I couldn't focus. So, I left my viewing chair and paced as I rehashed my recent fight.

First I cried at our mutual behavior. Then, I fumed. I built a case against my foe and layered it with past arguments.

I found the pattern, and while the themes were not fresh, my response was new: I had fought back. With cell phone to my ear, I yelled at her. And while the hot exchange left me exhausted, I was glad I had held my ground, gone toe-to-toe with my tough opponent.

This experience spurred me to review my squabbling style, as well as the one I had witnessed in my childhood. I propped two pillows on my bed, stretched out, and let the file tape flow across my brain.

In my 2006 memoir, "The Division Street Princess," I wrote this about my parents' quarrels: "Whenever I heard their arguments, I'd duck for cover, like a recruit frightened of battle. And although the two of them never came to blows and seemed to recuperate quickly, my wounds took longer to heal."

Forgive me for the marketing, but I just love that sentence. I believe it was this early experience that led me to the style I chose for my first marriage. I was determined to not repeat those painful scenes, so when I felt injured by my husband's actions, I chose silence. I stewed; complained to friends, let my children fight my battles -- anything to not engage. And so, during our 30-year-marriage, the two of us constructed a wall. Tiff-by-tiff, the bricks grew taller and more impenetrable with each year, until it toppled in divorce.

In comparison, my second marriage was a pleasure cruise.

We sailed along -- watching the same TV programs, walking our dog, taking occasional vacations -- and on the rare instances we argued, it was always Tommy who said, "Let's not be mad at each other. Let's talk about it."

A few words, maybe a tear from each of us, hugs, and then it was over.

I remember once, when my first husband was at our house -- gratefully, we had stayed friendly through the divorce and in the subsequent years, and Tommy enjoyed his company -- my second husband and I began to squabble. I can't remember what the issue was, but we tapped lightly, as if we were first-time kids in the ring.

"Why couldn't we have done that?" my first husband had said, as he watched Tommy and I tussle, and then make up quickly.

He was wistful as he asked this, and at the time, I answered, "I have no idea." But I do: my parents' union had infiltrated that first marriage and successfully silenced me.

Was husband #1 jealous that I had landed in a stable second marriage, or was he wondering it could've been different if I had only learned how to fight?

It isn't as if he and I hadn't booked therapy appointments way back then, where each on our own time would spill our secrets, our unhappiness, and our frustrations. But somehow, those scholarly souls couldn't solve our problems, and so after our three-decade marriage and a six-year separation, we signed the divorce papers.

After my most recent clash with the dear one, I pondered how I had journeyed from watching on the sidelines in my childhood, to righteous silence in my first marriage, to simple taps in my second, and finally, to the loud-mouthed, hotheaded battler I had become. Was it age that had toughened me, a conviction I was the injured party, or a desire to see only what I wanted to see?

It's likely my opponent and I will take a few days to lick our wounds. We'll kvetch to friends about the other's stubbornness. Then hopefully, we'll edge our way back towards each other, and to love.

THERAPY

The door was locked, so I took a seat on the floor opposite the office of my new therapist. Because I was early, I wasn't unsettled about my blocked entry; and I resisted taking it as a sign that this latest round of soul scrutiny was off to a bad start.

However, if she (let's call her Sarah) didn't arrive by my appointed time, then I would rise, dust myself off, and chalk it off to evidence that therapy need not be a weekly calendar notation.

But a few minutes before the hour, Sarah appeared -- breathless because she had ridden over on her bike. She apologized for the locked door and I was speedily ushered into a room that felt as familiar as a childhood bedroom.

There was the three-cushioned couch in a subtle grey and floral pattern, the side table with a box of Kleenex and bottles of water, landscapes and other serene artworks on the walls, a facing armchair in matching upholstery, with its own side table of clock and notepad.

In my 76 years of life, I have turned to therapy a handful of times. My slim record is not because I disdain the practice or am reluctant to reveal my secrets. Au contraire, I love therapy! Fifty-five minutes focused on me, a sympathetic witness to my angst, a collaborator in my version of the story; who wouldn't relish the experience.

All of my sessions were jump-started by a query. Some visits continued weekly for nearly a year; others curtailed in a few months.

Sondra (fictitious, too, but interestingly, all of my therapists' names did begin with the letter "S") was my first, sometime in the late '80s.

I was lured to Sondra through an article she had written about weight issues. I was a perpetual dieter, and thought Sondra could help me untangle my eating issues and enable me to drop 10 pounds.

But somehow during the very first session, our theme veered from my heft to my marriage, both of which were affecting my happiness. I can still see Sondra from those long ago days. She was wearing a loose-fitting tunic top and matching long skirt. *Shrink wear,* I thought at the time, *flowing, unrestricted, the better to encourage comfort and open dialogue.*

I discontinued therapy when my marriage improved (I still had the extra 10 pounds), but returned after my husband's surprise leave-taking in 1990. I went solo for a few sessions, he joined me for one, and despite Sondra being charmed with him, my spouse had his foot determinedly out the door.

My next bout of therapy was with a woman we'll call Stella, and it was to her whom I would come back to over the coming years. Stella is regal, with salt-and-pepper hair, and dressed in the requisite draping wardrobe.

Our first round was very short term, perhaps only three visits. I had only one question: if I was so unhappy in the marriage, why was I still crying about its demise?

"You were married for 30 years, sadness is normal," she said, which satisfied my need for any further sessions.

I returned to Stella in 2009 after my second husband, Tommy, and I had been together for 13 years. "He's a jerk," I told her. "When we first married, he'd write me love letters, hide syrupy Post-it notes in my gym bag. Now, nothing, and on top of that, he says inappropriate things to strangers."

As our appointments and Tommy's odd behavior continued, something new was added to the mix: he lost his ability to speak. Stella suggested a visit to a neurologist, and that's how my husband's dreadful brain degeneration was diagnosed. Once I realized his unsettling symptoms matched the illness, I ended therapy and transitioned from puzzled wife to compassionate caregiver.

Before I left Chicago for Los Angeles at the end of 2014, I had a few more sessions with Stella. She listened as I questioned my motivation for the move, and like a professor watching a student puzzle out an unsolved math theory, she sat patiently while I tossed pros and cons.

My second appointment with my LA therapist, Sarah, began in a more traditional fashion. Her outer office door was unlocked, so I settled on a chair in the waiting room. Exactly at the appointed hour, she opened the door to her private space.

As I unleashed my backpack and removed my hat, and placed both on the cushion next to me, Sarah uncapped her pen and placed a notepad in her lap.

"So, here's my question this week," I began.

BEST OF BOTH WORLDS

I have been accused of being a dabbler -- someone who hops in and out of jobs, groups, and residences quicker than the average person.

Others have named my disorder a reaction to boredom, which involves a constant need for a new, challenging project.

Lately, I've named myself a "participatory journalist" like George Plimpton who recorded his various experiences from the point of view as an amateur -- but in my case, rookie.

I have no problem accepting these labels, although I especially like the last one, and because I have no regrets about my quick decisions.

Every job I've had, including salesperson at the Gap, specialist at the Apple Store (three months apiece), and press aide for a Chicago mayor, communications director for a school superintendent, and account supervisor for public relations firms (one year each) introduced me to new friends, challenging assignments, fresh skills, and most importantly, essay topics.

The same "no regrets" applies to all of the neighborhoods I have convinced my spouses to move into. In my first marriage of 30 years, we lived in 15 different apartments, condos, or homes. Dear Tommy, who had lived in the same house for 25 years before I wandered into his life, was schlepped to three homes in 14 years.

Since his death in 2012, I've lived in two different apartments, and now -- drum roll, please -- I'm ready to leave Los Angeles and return to Chicago.

So at lease end, I hope to move to an apartment in one of the high-rises in Lakeshore East, a location that will put this participatory journalist in the midst of the city's vibrancy and near friends and relatives -- some of whom could use support as they care for aging partners, or need a pal at their side for own medical procedures.

This reverse move may come as a surprise to my readers and to viewers of published photos, all of which praise Los Angeles. These examples of my delightful eight months here with family and celebrities are accurate; there was no exaggeration.

But, being the quick decision-maker that I proudly call myself, I recognize I'm better off in Chicago, a city much easier to navigate for an older woman who elects not to drive.

While my hometown does have its struggles, it has moved ahead on tough urban issues, such as a reliable and speedy public transit system, solutions for chronic homelessness, and creating a downtown viable for residents, college students, retail, and visitors. And then there's the pizza and hot dogs.

My decision doesn't mean I have flunked here, or have regrets about the cross-country move, for I have learned things about myself, which wouldn't have occurred if I hadn't done the shift.

For example, with a Metro senior citizen pass, I get to far-flung shopping centers and doctors' appointments. I find fulfillment by volunteering at a nonprofit agency, and by attending weekly Torah study. I have made a good friend -- another grandmother transplant -- who drives and shares her favorite L.A. highlights. And, I took a 6-week workshop on How to Write a Half-hour TV Comedy, completed an original pilot and a spec script, and gained a manager who continues to seek opportunities for me.

All of the above was accomplished relatively easy for a speed demon like myself, but the primary cause for my move to Los Angeles was much trickier. Because I had not lived in the same city as my daughters for 25 years, and since I was unfettered in Chicago (no husband, house, dog, car, debt), I thought the time was right to jump into their world.

It turns out that my daughters' whirlwind lives are already over-stuffed with career and family responsibilities. While they try to include me in as many events and gatherings as possible, I find myself insatiable. No matter how often I see them, it is never enough for me.

Trying to make up for lost decades, and likely attempting to fill the void left by Tommy's death, I turned needy and greedy -- features unbecoming to me and difficult for my beloved daughters.

But, instead of considering this decision an abandonment of Los Angeles, I'll add Bi-Coastal to my labels and have the best of both worlds. For special events and family celebrations, in harsh winter months, and when the itch for something fresh enters my brain, I'll return to the city of treasured children and grandchildren, temperate climes, and glitter.

And when my L.A. and Boston daughters book a visit to see both Chicago parents -- hopefully with grandchildren in tow -- they'll have my new playground as an attraction.

Just think of the essays that await us.

PACKING

The first thing I placed in the shipping box was a container with his ashes. It was lightweight because scoops had already been removed and scattered. One batch of my second husband's remains went to Jackson Park where Tommy got a hole in one. Another was spread among the plantings outside the YMCA, his longtime gym; and one more in the park where every morning for 12 years we walked our dog.

Next, I tucked in his watch and wallet -- both decades old because he thought it foolish to replace them. I slipped his wedding ring on the watchstrap, threaded it closed, and tucked it in.

Just as I was about to seal the box and affix a mailing label for Chicago, I heard, "I was wondering when you were going to get your butt home."

Tommy! My deceased spouse had decided to visit. "Get your butt home," he'd order when he was alive and I traveled away from him. He was teasing back then, and now for fun, repeating the phrase.

"I'm not surprised you're glad I'm returning to Chicago," I said, smiling as I resurrected his voice, which was clear rather than dimmed by his end-of-life aphasia. "You were never a fan of Los Angeles," I said. "Too spread out, horrible traffic, wasn't that your view?"

"Listen sweetheart," he said. "We both grew up in Chicago. We've got friends there we've known since childhood. That's not easy to replace."

My make-believe visitor was a clue it was time to take a break from packing. As I was about to continue with Tommy, another speaker seeped through my head.

"Remember I told you Princess, that I always wanted to live at State and Madison?" It was my dad who's been dead since 1958, but evidently eager to have a say. "I heard you're moving into a building downtown. Terrific; you're finally listening to me." He held a cigarette between two fingers, and when he saw my stare, said, "Carte blanche. No restrictions."

"We're happy you're returning to Chicago, too." This was a duet. "Mom, Dad!" I said to my former in-laws, a lovely couple that came with my first marriage. "This is the only time you've returned for a conversation since you died. Why now?"

"To be honest, we were very unhappy when you moved to Los Angeles, but it wasn't our place to pry." It was my father-in-law taking the lead. "Even though you divorced, we felt sure you'd be in Chicago, in our child's life forever, watching over each other."

My mother-in-law, ever the polite one, said, "When we learned you were moving back, and picked an apartment near our dear one, we just had to come and tell you how pleased we are."

Wow, this was getting to be some pow-wow! Just as I was about to respond, another speaker joined in. I was wondering when she was going to show up. "Am I the only one unhappy that you're leaving L.A. and my grandchildren and great-grandchildren?" she said. "I finally had you all in one place, and typical of you, you're on the move again."

I wasn't distressed by my mother's opinion; I was just happy to have the chance to conjure her vision. She died in 1981, still a beauty with hair barely touched by gray. Our kids were teens then, old enough for their talent to dazzle her.

"I knew it; I knew it, back in their high school years," she said. "I predicted they'd be remarkable. " She looked triumphant, as if she were on stage with her granddaughters, holding their hands as they accepted awards.

My in-laws soon leapt in. "Those girls are something else," they agreed, wanting to assure their DNA was also credited.

"Listen," I said to the celestial crowd. "I know you have differing opinions about my returning to Chicago." Four heads nodded. "But for now, I'd really appreciate it if you'd just watch over me and my move."

Tommy was the first to offer: "Since I'm the most recent up here, I'll be closest to your flight home. I've got that covered."

"No worries," Dad said. "I'll ride shotgun in the delivery trucks coming your way, just to make sure everything arrives on time."

"I suppose we can handle the reserved elevator," my father-in-law said. "Oh dear," from his wife. "Thirty-seventh floor. I suppose it'll be fine."

We waited for Mom to volunteer. "When all of the furniture is in place and you're finally in bed in your new home," she said. "I'll tuck you in."

Content now, I returned to my task and assembled another box, larger this time, to hold family photographs. Everyone was coming with.

BALCONIES, STAIRS, STOOPS, AND FOLDING CHAIRS

As the sun rises, I can peer to the east from the small balcony of my new 37th floor apartment and see Navy Pier.

A slight turn of the head to the west brings into view the Tribune Tower. The Chicago River, in its natural green tint, and Lake Michigan -- blue as far as the eye can see -- are also part of my sky-top view. It is quiet now; only the soft rush of early morning autos reaches my ears.

Sitting outdoors on a perfect Chicago summer day coaxes my mind to travel backwards to other unforgettable places where I have perched. And like a jigsaw puzzle whose picture only emerges when all of the parts are snuggly in place, I add the characters that help create a picture of my past.

The year is 1996, early evening; I am sitting at the top of a long staircase outside my Henderson St. townhouse. My Golden Retriever, Sasha, is hip-to-hip next to me. She rises and madly rushes to the bottom stair to greet her friend: it is our neighbor Tommy returning from work.

As Tommy pets Sasha, I boldly ask, "If you ever want to catch a movie, let me know." I have practiced this sentence because dog and I have said good morning to this fella ever since we moved in. He'd be out for a run the same time as Sasha's first walk. I had learned he was about my age and single. At the time, I was merely looking for a pal in my young neighborhood, and thought Tommy a candidate.

"I go to the Y Mondays, Wednesdays, and Fridays," he said, likely eager to add his fitness credentials. So any Tuesday or Thursday." I picked a Tuesday, and that was how my second marriage began.

Now, let's flip the calendar backwards to 1970. See my 32-year-old self as I sit on the stoop of a townhouse in South Commons on Chicago's near south side. The brick homes are built around a square, so my neighbor and I can lounge, and at the same time watch our children at play. My daughters are six and seven-and-a-half years old, my friend's two daughters nearly the same.

The scene looks idyllic: the children scooting and whooping in the courtyard are shades of white, black, and brown.

We live in a community where that palette was the purpose -- urban pioneers, eager to be part of an experiment to learn if people of different races, incomes, and ages could live together.

While the youngsters are carefree, these two mothers are dour, for we are both in first marriages chipping at the edges. "I don't know what to do," I tell my friend. "Is divorce the answer?" I have asked the question, but I stay wed until we part many years later.

Now let's travel far back and ride a Red Hornet streetcar to Division Street circa 1940's Chicago. It's not me on outdoor seats; instead my parents and neighbors on this immigrant block.

"Lock up," my mother says to my father. She is talking about Irv's Finer Foods, our corner grocery store. She has removed and folded the apron she wears in the store and hid it behind the counter where she will unhappily unfold it tomorrow and place it over her head. She does this carefully, so as not to mess her upswept hair.

"Some kids might want an ice cream bar," my father the askew optimist says. He is sitting on a folding chair outside of the store. His cronies are lined up on one side and my mother on the other. He puts his hand on her bare arm -- it is a hot summer's night -- and she shakes it away. The movement is her answer and a gesture that cracks my heart.

Dad ignores the slight and turns to his pal. "Did you listen to the Cubs game?" he says. His brown eyes catch the light of the lampposts. "*Farshtunken*," his friend slams. "They're still my boys," my father says.

While our parents are lined up on the chairs they have schlepped from closets, my brother and I, and a slapdash mix of kids are racing wildly on the concrete sidewalk. "Oley Oley Ocean free," someone screams. "You're it!" shouts another.

Before I leave my balcony and reminiscing, I wonder, *why these scenes and not others.* Surely there were patios and porches where I enjoyed the summer air and dear companions. But when I peer into each vignette, I realize they were all wrapped in beginnings and endings: A sweetheart married and buried. A young love found and lost. A childhood carefree and sad.

Life.

IMPOSTER

I'm confused about the name of the dog nuzzling me nose to nose. Is this Pippin, Rosie, Enzo or Ellie?

There's at least six of these small breeds: Shih Tzus, Pugs, Beagles, Spaniels, Terriers, Cockapoos, and mixes of them all, that wander the dog park and eventually wind up on my lap.

While I fancy the larger dogs -- the Goldens, Labradors, and blends of the two -- these big guys are like adolescents, racing after each other, wrestling a bit, and then resuming their manic chasing.

"Which is yours?" The question came from a fairytale blond seated next to me on the bench. While she waited for my answer, her eyes tracked the tiny mounds of grass, trees, and ponds, ready to coo when I pointed out my pet.

I hesitated a bit, and then confessed, "Um, I don't have a dog." I said this quietly for I didn't want the word to spread that I was an imposter, someone pretending to have a pet and worse, possibly planning to snatch one.

"I just moved into the building a week ago," I quickly added, "and don't have a pet. But, I've had Golden Retrievers in the past and miss being around dogs." What I didn't say -- because I wanted to avoid pity or solutions -- was that my budget couldn't squeeze in bills for vet, dog food, or boarding during planned trips to Los Angeles. Those details could wait.

This must've mollified her, because she then introduced me to a bench friend, and pets. "That's Enzo and my Ellie," she said. At the sound of their names, the two dogs paused briefly in their rounds, lifted their button-sized ears, glanced toward their owners, and then renewed their mini trots.

My plot was working. I remembered how my two dogs swiftly introduced me to friends in new neighborhoods, so I was trying it again, but this time, without my own furry one in the crowd. I knew that dog owners are drawn to each other like long-lost relatives. Instead of DNA, the bond is affection and addiction to animals.

But as I think of it, there was one dog-induced friendship that didn't go smoothly. The time was 1990; I was 52 and separated from my husband of 30 years. While a bit sad at the split, I was also giddy because I relished the fresh freedom. "I eat pizza on the couch while watching TV," I told friends, which at the time seemed the epitome of new beginnings.

With my Golden Retriever, Sasha, I met -- let's call her Lauren -- and her dog Midnight. (Not his real name either.)

She was likely 20 years younger than I, but we bonded because we were single women with dogs.

Lauren and I met daily. We walked our dogs together. We visited each other's homes. We sat on bare and carpeted floors to continue our conversations and simultaneously stroke our pets. We were best friends. Then David entered the picture. (Of course, fictitious name.)

I had met David at a singles event and was immediately beguiled because he was the opposite of my husband. David smoked small cigars and pot, drove fast, ate revolting food, and was into New Age philosophy. And because I was feeling like a kid released from a long, intense residency in a boarding school, all of this made me aflutter.

Now, one of David's proclivities that I didn't include in the above line-up was that he related easily to women. Because of that, he had many female fans that relished his heart-to-heart conversations.

Lauren became one of them. "We're only friends," she said, when I claimed discomfort about their intense relationship. David seconded, "You have no reason to be jealous."

But their words didn't appease; I coveted their intimacy. Eventually, I wrote a long -- quite excellent and well-reasoned -- letter to the both of them, breaking off my bonds. They protested I was off base, but neither chose me over the other.

Now that I consider that time with Lauren and David, I wonder who was the imposter in that dog-engendered relationship? Was it Lauren posing as my friend so she could snuggle with David? Was it David believing his female friendships wouldn't evolve into something more? Or was it I, in a pseudo romance where I pretended to embrace David's unhealthy and risky lifestyle, but in truth rejected it?

Okay, I'll cop to being a bit of a fraud 35 years ago, but today in this dog park, I'm not trying to fool anyone: Bring on the pooches.

ABANDONMENT ISSUES

The super thick exercise mat won't arrive until tomorrow. But I'm hyped up to begin, so I improvise. Two curly bathroom rugs tease. I place one on top of the other and plop them on the hallway floor.

From my filing cabinet -- um, a cardboard box stored in a closet -- I retrieve a folder labeled, Medical Soloway. Did I place my physical therapy exercises here, or could I have tossed them in my recent move?

Found! Now, I have no excuse to ignore the suggestion from my internist that began with her question: "Does the pain start in the butt and radiate to your leg?"

"Exactly," I had said during a consultation the previous day. Was she clairvoyant, I wondered, or had a glance at my online chart revealed this was a recurring symptom?

"I've booked an appointment late in September for an epidural injection," I said. "Those shots helped in the past."

I went on, "The pain started after walking at least a mile." But instead of congratulating me for my daily treks as I had hoped, she announced, "sciatica."

Then she turned from the computer screen and said, "Actually, physical therapy may be better for sciatica than undergoing the needle."

As she was reaching for a prescription pad, I confessed, "Um, I did six weeks of PT in Los Angeles."

Her face brightened, "Did it help?"

"While I was doing it," I said.

"Well, perhaps you should try again before the epidural," she said. "Let the surgeon know the results and perhaps you can avoid the shot."

That was the conversation that had me flat on my back, with stomach muscles pulled tight, and counting to 10 with each stretch. After the last maneuver, compressing on the two rugs, I scolded myself for abandoning these beneficial exercises.

If they were indeed easing the pain encountered with long walks, why did I shove the instructions deep into the file cabinet and ditch a padded mat in the L.A. apartment I recently left? I wondered: why are good intentions so easily dumped?

Instead of remaining on the duo mat to ponder the question, I retreated to my bed, the better to meditate on my latest desertion. With my eyes closed and the sliding door open to a morning breeze and the sounds of early traffic, I retraced other worthwhile plans I had promised to pursue, but instead paused.

Let's see, there were courses on speaking Spanish beyond the present tense, lessons on swimming while breathing on either side, private piano lessons so I could play Rogers and Hart, and group singing classes to accompany myself.

The most enjoyable part of all of these activities -- including my recent physical therapy -- was the pre-research and purchases. There might be new workbooks, wardrobes, equipment, and other necessities.

And once an instructor and location were determined, came the exquisite next step of entering the details on electronic and paper calendars. Ever the optimist, each activity would be "a recurring event," which I would optimistically stretch out for an entire semester.

Oh stop it. I know you're imagining I flunked at all of those endeavors, threw out the workbooks, tossed the goggles, sold the piano, and cursed the composers. Well, no, nothing so abrupt or dramatic. Each one slowly slipped away, like a full moon that disappears from the sky.

If friends or family inquired as to the status of any pursuit, I'd say, "I just got too busy with work and couldn't fit it in any more." (Substitute "lazy," "bored," or "discouraged" and you'd be closer to the truth.)

Fortunately, I barely remember the tails of my attempts, but I easily recall the beginnings. So, after a year's time, when a fresh catalog appears in my mailbox, or when a new apartment offers both an indoor and outdoor pool, or when a promotional flyer is pasted on a nearby bulletin board, I feel the familiar lures of "Why Not?"

Of course, doing daily physical therapy exercises doesn't exactly match the pleasures I would win if I were to *hablo español,* do laps, tinkle the ivories, or croon. On the other hand, if I performed them every morning without fail, it's possible I could walk a mile without returning home for an

Advil, heating pad, or icepack. And perhaps I could cancel the epidural.

And, if I were able to repair my body and walk or trot without stabs, perhaps I could one day run a marathon. Hold on; let me look into that.

MEAN GIRL

So far this month, two people are mad at me -- wait, maybe three. Perhaps even you?

Surprisingly, I'm okay with that. In my advancing age I've decided to switch from a lifetime of Nice Girl to an occasional Mean Girl.

You won't find me tripping the feeble, or hurling insults at strangers; just that I may do something that makes you mad -- like acting haughty or telling you *no* -- and, I can live with that.

This recent decision is *so* liberating! It all began in discussions with several acquaintances and I was not able to satisfy either with my *No, can't do* response.

While my repeated *No* eventually terminated the dialogues, it didn't stop my brain from simmering. Because of my decades of being nice, polite, and diffident, I couldn't leave the issues as settled. Instead, I obsessed about my dissenting and anticipated a night of tossing.

It was then the refreshing idea slipped in among my turbulent thoughts: *It's okay for someone to not like me, or to be mad at me; I will survive.*

And with that light bulb moment, I felt unburdened, and knew I could then sleep peacefully.

Of course, this liberating notion required a bit of research: When did my intent of being Nice Girl begin? So while visions of avengers skipped on by without pausing, calendar years flipped backwards until I reached childhood.

I see pre-teen me posing in front of a three-way mirror in a department store circa 1950. Mother is seated on a cushion surveying the outfit I am sampling. "You look fine," she says, responding to my dour expression.

I dearly love this beautiful woman who is scrutinizing my fashion show. With her upswept hairdo, blue eyes, Max Factor red lipstick, and beauty queen shape, she resembles a film star.

She is adorned with costume jewelry, a sweater I wish had a higher neckline, a slim skirt, and high heels she insists on despite the resulting bunions.

The scene in this department store is familiar: My mother selects my clothes. As usual, I button my lip about my hatred of her choices because I believe my tie to her so fragile that I dare not oppose. "If you want me to get it," I say about each unappealing ensemble, "let's do it."

So Nice Daughter continued until Mother died. She left this earth without ever learning of my loathing of the bulky winter storm coat, the school shoes with thick heels, or the faux cashmere sweaters that made my skin itch. I can live with that; she didn't deserve to ever meet Mean Girl.

Nice Girl was also Nice Student; first to raise her hand, turn in her perfect penmanship paper, and volunteer to erase the black board. That's why the unpleasant time in the assembly hall still reproduces darkly whenever I try to recall my eight years at Lafayette Elementary.

"I can't see the stage," I said to my chum on my left as I tapped the stiff cotton of her blouse. "Can I try on your glasses?"

After Sandy handed them to me and I placed them atop my nose and ears, I let out, "Wow, I can even see the buckles on their shoes."

"Elaine, stop talking or you'll have to leave the assembly," said Miss Lowe, her finger touching her lips for emphasis.

This had never happened to Nice Girl! I removed my friend's glasses, handed them to her, and used my small arm to wipe tears. I was mortified. In my childish mind, that incident dumped me into the group of bad kids, those who would be sent to the principal's office.

I had made the teacher I adored mad at me, and that incident must've seeped into my brain and stuck there as if it were chewed gum on the bottom of an unlucky shoe.

History reveals that my desire to prevent anyone's displeasure went beyond those I care about. I see now that it protected everyone from Mean Girl, like an insurance policy that promises full coverage even in the event of flood or earthquake.

As I look back on these petty examples of how important it was for me to be Nice, I wonder how off base I had been. Perhaps Mother would've taken my view, considered it, and said, "Oh, I never realized that. Of course, you can choose what you like."

And maybe Miss Lowe, if she had known how her simple shushing had devastated me and left a lifelong stain, would've pulled me aside and said something like, "I know this was not your usual behavior. You're still my star pupil."

No matter. *You've* been warned: Watch out for Mean Girl.

PIANO

The freight elevator is reserved for Friday between 10 and noon. A member of the maintenance crew has already been to my apartment and removed from a hallway closet two folding doors and wire shelving.

For my part, I've shifted its contents to a different closet in my 582-square-foot studio apartment. Soon, a pre-owned Everett Upright Piano, with bench, will occupy that empty area, which once housed a handful of sweaters, a mat for morning stretches, a pail, broom, and dry mop. Instead of a wave of a hand like some ordinary wizard, I have used wit and brawn to transform a once humble space into a music room.

"How long have you been playing?" the eager salesman had asked as we climbed two flights of stairs to review pianos in my price range.

Catching my breath, I had said, "Oh, I can't really play. I'm a perpetual beginner. All I want is to learn how to play Rogers and Hart." He hesitated, perhaps wondering if I was serious in my search, then shrugged *whatever* and continued up another flight.

I didn't think he needed the history of my piano quest, but I'll tell you: Neither my first husband nor I played, but because we believed a house filled with music was a bonus, in 1970 we bought an upright and offered lessons to our daughters.

From the moment six-year-old Faith sat down on the bench; she treated the instrument as if it were her long-lost twin. (Her sister, Jill, tried lessons, but quickly decided to leave that particular talent to her sibling.)

My draw to the piano didn't occur during those years; it wasn't until another time and place that I decided to take lessons. It was the '80s, and the upright had been exchanged for an ebony baby grand. I can still see that handsome piece, with its wing-shaped lid, which seemed to send its notes soaring.

I wish I could remember the name of the young man who was my first teacher, and led me through Alfred's Basic Adult Piano Course - Level 1. But in 1990, when my first marriage ended, the baby grand and lessons exited, too.

Tommy and I first met in 1996, and we learned we had the same favorite song: Rogers' and Hart's "It Never Entered My Mind." That commonality, plus others, led to marriage and another piano.

I was never able to smoothly play *our* tune, but I could pick my way through George Gershwin's, "They Can't Take That Away From Me."

I can still see -- and hear -- my wannabe crooner standing at the side of our Yamaha, belting out "*The way your wear your hat...*" Like an aged nightclub duo, I'd I search for the right keys while my sweetheart patiently waited for me to catch up to his lyrics.

After Tommy died in 2012, I sold our house. The piano went, too, as part of an estate sale. Because I was moving to a studio apartment in River North, I believed there'd be no room for the instrument. Or, maybe I thought any images of our schmaltzy showbiz scene would be too hard to bear.

During my nine-month stay in Los Angeles, my roomy one-bedroom apartment could've housed a piano, even a baby grand, but I never desired one. It wasn't until I returned to Chicago, and in a conversation with a friend that the thought came up. I must've been gloomy the day of our lunch, because she advised: "Find something to make you happy."

Happy. Then, clear as day I heard Tommy's tenor: "*The way you haunt my dreams, no, no, they can't take that away from me.*" I saw the two of us in the dining room alcove where the upright stood. I heard us laugh as I struggled with chords.

"A piano," I told my friend. "A piano and lessons; that made me happy."

So, once the pre-owned Everett comes home, and I hang portraits of jazz giants on walls where wire once hung, I plan to host "Sing Along Sundays." By then, I'll have purchased a few songbooks and those who can squeeze in, and are willing to play piano, or sing, will bring alive Rogers, Hart, Gershwin, and others of that era.

During those times, perhaps our chorus will imagine ourselves in a favorite musical. And because my mind's eye knows no limits, I'll see Tommy there, too.

Maybe by then, I'll be adept at our favorite song, and I can accompany him as he sings, "*And wish that you were there again, to get into my hair again, it never entered my mind.*"

BAD GRANDMA

We are sitting knee-to-knee at the top of a long flight of stairs that runs from the first floor of my daughter's Los Angeles home, to the second. There are three bedrooms up here; two are empty -- the adults having left for the night. And the third, where my 6-year-old grandson was supposed to be slumbering, has just been vacated.

"Call Mommy and tell her to come home," he says, one hand on the banister and the other wiping fresh tears from his face.

"No, I'm not," I say. "Mommy needs a night out."

His tears, which I believe are as false as those of a screen idol, slide from a trickle to full faucet. I am impressed with this talent.

"I want Mommy," he repeats.

"I can put you to bed," I say. After all, I had already fulfilled the prescription left by his mother: We cuddled under the covers, I flipped the pages of a favorite book and read dramatically -- playing all of the characters in different tones of voices -- and, I kissed his sweet forehead before twirling the light knob off and slipping out the door.

"Call Daddy. Call Isaac. Call Faith," he said. His father, brother, aunt; I waited for him to add the postman, gardener, housekeeper -- anyone but bad Grandma.

"I don't feel safe," he said, tossing a grenade. I smiled as I heard a sentence likely gleaned from kindergarten warnings.

"What can I do to make you feel safe?"

"Call Mommy."

"You're acting like a bully," I said. My grandson paused his tears for a bit and turned to look at me. He couldn't believe his ears, and his luck.

"You shouldn't call me a bully," he said. "That's not allowed at school."

I could see the scoreboard in my head, and his hometown team was trouncing the visiting one. Then, came my next foul: I started to cry. Not false tears as I believed my grandson was producing, and not sobs, just wet whispers of defeat.

"You win," I said. We had been at this for 30 minutes and I was ready to wave the white flag. "Let's go downstairs and call your mother."

When we reached the guest room where I was spending the night, he hopped in my bed, smiling as if he had been designated Most Valuable Player.

My cell phone had already received a text from my daughter. "How did everything go?" she wrote. "Were you able to put him to sleep?"

Self-pity turned to pique. My second born -- the recipient of decades of my love and devotion -- had predicted I'd encounter difficulty in putting her own second born to bed.

She knew I was fresh at this, having lived in different cities for all of his young years. Why had she not warned me? Why had she allowed me to enter the game like a player without proper headgear?

I returned her text: "I failed. He wants you home."

"On my way," she sent back.

When I turned to tell him the good news, he was fast asleep on my bed. His mother arrived, shook her head, and then carried him upstairs.

The next morning, my grandson and I greeted each other warily. Instead of pouting, I opted to put the previous night's episode behind me. "What would you like for breakfast?" I asked, kissing the top of his head. "We have Cheerios, or if you prefer, waffles." I was acting Diner Waitress in a game we often played.

"Cheerios," he said, evidently also eager to erase our evening dust-up.

The next day after I returned to my Los Angeles apartment, my daughter phoned. "He said you called him a bully and that you cried."

"True and true," I said.

"You shouldn't have done either," she said.

"I was unprepared," I said. "I didn't plan my reaction and couldn't help my tears."

"You're the adult," she said. "You should've known better."

My shoulders sunk as I felt another round slipping away. "I'm sorry," I said. "I wish it had turned out differently."

That evening, I sent my daughter a text. "How about I come over early tomorrow and give him breakfast? You can sleep in."

"That would be lovely," she typed back. We were not opponents after all. Obviously, the three of us had regretted our actions, words, and wounds, but remain deeply attached.

Now, because my daughter is an award-winning TV writer and director, the unfortunate scene just described could possibly be fictionalized and turn up in one of her episodes. Luckily, I can first describe it here, from my POV.

So score one for grandmas -- good, bad, and somewhere in between.

SANCTUARY

I slipped into an aisle seat figuring I could sneak out early if I got bored, or if I felt out of place. I looked up as others entered the synagogue's sanctuary and I'd nod a greeting when I'd spot a familiar face. As a pianist struck up notes and a choir of four began to sing prayers for the Friday night service, I settled in.

But why, in the midst of this fellowship and serenity, did I feel as guilty as if I had crept into a casino?

I was embarrassed to tell friends and family of my evening activity because upon returning to Chicago from Los Angeles three months ago, I had declared: "I've given up religion. I'm not going to High Holiday services this year or join a synagogue."

My dear crowd accepted this decision without debate because they have been witness to my forays in and out of Judaism. Growing up in the 1940's, my family's relationship with religion was cultural, rather than observant: We devoured fatty foods; championed Jewish athletes, movie stars, and comedians; supported Israel; and prayed that headlined criminals were not part of our tribe. And we attended synagogue services only once a year on the High Holidays.

But that mediocre piety didn't prevent my parents from pushing my brother Ron to become a Bar Mitzvah. As for me, in 1951, when I was 13 -- the age for this rite of passage -- girls in my group weren't similarly coerced. So I faltered on my faith for several decades.

Things changed in 1989, and I peg it on Empty Nest Syndrome. Both of our daughters were out of the house and I was seeking a project my spouse and I could do together. Instead of moving to a new residence -- which was my usual solution for our feeble marriage -- I suggested we join a synagogue.

We did. I jumped in, submerged, and resurfaced with a desire to have an adult Bat Mitzvah. I hired a tutor, learned to read Hebrew for my Torah portion, chanted, and hosted a celebration. Alas, one year later, our marriage expired and my link to that Reconstructionist synagogue ended, too.

In 2012, after my second husband Tommy died and I moved from our house to a downtown apartment, I joined a Reform synagogue where on Saturday mornings a group of 20 or so debated the week's Torah portion. "I love the intellectual stimulation," I told those skeptical of this fresh trail in my religious journey.

In Los Angeles, I quickly found another Reform temple and another series of Saturday morning studies. So why, after these two seemingly worthy religious experiences, did

I vow, upon returning home to Chicago, that I would be avoiding Judaism, Torah study, and the High Holidays?

"I wanted to feel part of a community," I told a friend, whining like a pathetic teenager who had been excluded from the popular girls' clique. "But I was never invited to anyone's home for dinner. At both synagogues, they'd all been together for decades, and evidently weren't interested in squeezing in this newcomer."

"Maybe if you had stayed longer," she suggested, "or joined committees, then you'd feel more part of the group." But I wanted to be immediately bonded. I was impatient, felt wounded, and decided I was finished with religion.

So, what happened last Friday to send me to evening services at the very same Chicago Reform temple I had huffed my way out of? My theory is while I originally believed I was seeking community and intellectual stimulation, I was really searching for something deeper, something to heal losses. In the first case, I was a recent widow who had buried a dear husband, and in the second, a transplant who moved away from good friends in a beloved city.

Evidently some pains remain: Tommy's death still feels fresh. And by returning to Chicago, I left behind my adored Los Angeles family. Add some in my circle face health challenges. Perhaps it is these facts of life that propelled me to find a harbor.

At last Friday night's service, as I sat in the synagogue's sanctuary, I listened to the choir and absorbed the rabbi's words. (In my absence, a new rabbi and assistant rabbi came on board. The latter is a woman -- a bonus in my view). And, I joined the congregation in reciting communal prayers for healing and mourning.

Based on my seesaw history with Judaism, my relatives and friends may be skeptical about this current religious plunge and wonder how long it will last.

Does it matter?

SHRINKING

I had three choices: I could drag over the stepstool that was across the aisle, climb to the highest shelf, and reach up and snatch the bottle of house brand Vinegar and Oil salad dressing. Or I could wander the supermarket to uncover a clerk. Maybe, I could catch the first tall person I'd see and plead for help.

Because I'm prone to disaster scenarios, I envisioned bitty me atop the stool, losing my footing, hanging onto the shelf itself, hauling it and its contents down with me, and falling flat into a sea of Caesar, Italian, and Ranch.

Instead, I chose option three and called out to a man who entered the aisle: "Tall person!"

He pointed to his chest, indicating he was unsure if I was referring to him, or if he had encountered a demented elder mistaking him for a wayward son.

"Could you get that bottle of salad dressing?" I said, pointing upward and smiling to make sure he understood my mirth. "I'm horizontally challenged."

With the ease of a basketball player, he put one hand around the neck of my prey and handed it to me. "No problem," he said, likely relieved I was sane.

Such episodes describe the life of an adult under five feet tall and shrinking. The towering supermarket shelf is just one inconvenience we wee ones endure. The other side includes the adjectives assigned to our stature. For example, this scene in the women's locker room at a former health club: I was at the mirror, putting on makeup, nude except for a towel around my torso. She was to my right, smiling down at me. A tall woman, five ten, I'd guess.

"You're so cute!" she had said. "How tall <u>are</u> you?"

I shifted to the left; afraid she might next pat my head, as if I were a puppy or toddler. "I used to be four eleven and a half, but now I'm four nine," I said. "You shrink as you get older." As soon as the words left my mouth, images of Dorothy's Wicked Witch rode into my brain. Instead of a broomstick, I saw the crone dissolve into a puddle with only her pointy hat remaining.

I suppose I should be used to cuddly responses to my height by now. After all, I'm 77, and have always been the shortest in a group. Early class photos are evidence: first row, first seat, and feet barely touching the floor.

"You were so cute," that's how my best friend Ruth remembers me in sixth grade when we first met. "Just like a doll." We have been close friends for more than 60 years. Ruth says she's shrinking, too, but she's still at least five nine.

I don't remember it bothering me in grade school, but I think by high school the words started to chafe, and the older I got, the more irritating "cute" and "doll" became. If it were up to me, I'd select comments about my personality, not my dimensions.

To be honest, I 've never felt handicapped as a short woman. I do my best work sitting, where size is irrelevant. Yes, I have to perch on a phone book to get my hair shampooed, and I have a hard time at the movies if someone tall fills the seat in front. And, there's that supermarket thing.

Now that I think of it, one reason I fell for my first husband, who at six feet proposed despite my size, was because he thought me smart, clever, and funny. As for me, I loved his tallness – believing I had gained stature, just by hanging on his arm.

But from the beginning there were problems with our differences in altitudes. "Can't hear you," I'd shout up as we held hands walking down the street. And when we danced, his arm around my shoulder, my nose at his navel, we were comic.

My sweetheart of a second husband was a perfect five seven. No communication or waltz snags. While he did throw in a few "you're so cute" endearments, I knew it was my accomplishments he bragged about to friends.

I've been a widow for three years now, and am thinking I'd like a male companion -- not a husband, just a buddy for early dinners, TV watching, and chaste spooning. If he's somewhere in my age range, his height has likely dipped a few inches, too. Fortunately, for the three activities I've just identified, that shouldn't be a problem.

RENEWED

It takes three pillows to lift me high enough to see above the Kia Soul's dashboard. "I had great visibility in my last car, a Honda Fit," I tell Michelle, as she hauls a trio from the trunk. "I'll be more confident if I can see both front fenders."

"Pedestrians, too," Michelle says, "you have to watch out for pedestrians and bicyclists. Check left, front, and right before proceeding or turning, think 'left, front, and right.'"

I repeat, "Left, front, and right," hoping her mantra will guarantee that any walkers and riders in my path remain unscathed.

Michelle, who is young enough to be a granddaughter, has picked me up at 6:00 in the morning for my first driving lesson. After two hours of instruction and practice, she will accompany me to the DMV, lead me through the lines, and then wait while a tester takes over the passenger seat.

It was just four months ago, on my 77th birthday, when I decided to let my driver's license expire. I reasoned that since I hadn't driven for nearly two years, I wouldn't bother with the renewal and instead apply for a state identification card. After all, with my two legs, shared rides -- Uber and Lyft -- and the CTA, I had competently managed my travel needs.

Recently, the lack of a license started to nag: I felt my decision to forgo renewal had prematurely aged me. And the only way to reverse that discomfort was to get it back. But, first I'd had to pass a road test.

I was certain any licensed friend would be willing to escort me to the DMV, and then turn over their car for the test, but I was too skittish for that route. If I could take a few lessons from an accredited driving school, and then use their auto for the road test, I was certain my chances of passing would improve.

A search on Yelp led me to the Nova Driving School, to Michelle, and to the three pillows between my tush and the Kia's front seat.

In 1952, when my dad first taught me how to drive, I pulled pillows from our plastic-covered sofa to prop me in his four-door Buick. As he flicked ashes from Camels into the butt-littered tray, he showed me how to grasp the wheel in the ten and two positions, execute the hand-over-hand turn, operate the stick shift, and play the clutch.

And he divulged secrets to parallel parking, which I have since passed down to two daughters and one grandson: Line up your car with one that is parked at the curb. Slowly, back up into the empty space as you turn the steering wheel to the right. Fix your eyes on the right headlight of the car parked behind. Aim for your target, then reverse the direction of the steering wheel. Slip in.

"Make a left at the next light," Michelle says. I push the lever down to signal my turn, step gently on the brake, and come to a neat stop at the red signal. My instructor looks pleased as I say, "left, front, and right" while checking each of the three directions.

"You've got this," Michelle says, likely relieved that despite my age and lack of practice for two years; she will not have to stomp on her instructor's brake.

"You haven't forgotten anything."

"This is fun," I say, resisting the urge to floor the gas pedal as if I were a felon fleeing the scene. Muscle memory has renewed and I am once again the teenager who has been handed the keys to the Buick.

"Both hands on the wheel," Michelle orders, after my left dropped to my lap following the classic hand-over-hand.

"But that's how I always drive," I tell her.

"You could lose a point for that," she says.

When Dad drove, he used only one hand for the wheel; the left lingered out the rolled down window. His arm was tanned from finger to elbow, and the remainder white as his grocery store apron.

During the road test, I forced myself to keep both hands on the wheel. And with Michelle's meticulous instructions, and memories of my Dad's lessons, I easily passed. Sadly, I wasn't required to parallel park; I would've aced that.

To keep fresh, I'll occasionally rent a Zipcar, haul pillows from my couch, and take a spin. Anyone need a lift? Costco run?

HAVE PILLOWS, WILL TRAVEL

My lifelong friend Ruth is allowing me to practice driving in her 2003 green Honda Accord. "I have to be able to see over the steering wheel," I tell her. She raises the driver's seat as high as it can go.

I remove two pillows from my shopping bag, place them on the seat, and then hop atop. "Not yet," I say, balling up my puffy jacket, and adding it to the small tower.

"Perfect," I say.

I turn on the ignition, and pull out of the parking lot of Calo Restaurant and into Clark St. en route to Ruth's condo in Evanston. This will be my first time at a wheel, after just passing the road test a week ago and renewing my license. Gratefully, I am at ease. I had owned Hondas for most of my adult life and although it has been more than two years since I drove any car, I feel at home.

But, this was not how the day was supposed to go. Instead of Ruth's Honda, I had planned to drive a spiffy red 2015 VW Golf from the garage of the Sheraton Hotel to our restaurant meeting place. I picked the Golf from the rental agency's website because I wanted a hatchback with rear seats that fold down and offer extra visibility for backing up.

I was desperate to have my first drive go smoothly, so on Monday, the day before my Tuesday reservation; I played the role of a bank robber casing the joint. First, I clocked the time it would take to walk from my apartment to the hotel -- 10 minutes.

After twirling through the revolving door, I studied my printed instructions: "Go to level P1. Walk out of the waiting area and you will see our cars along the north wall."

My quarry -- as precious as a safe filled with treasury bonds -- was a standout among the bland sedans along the wall.

Outside the hotel, I located the exit from the garage, and then recited "left on Park St., right on Illinois, follow the cars to Lake Shore Drive, exit on Foster, right on Clark St., left to Calo parking lot." (I had debated taking surface streets rather than the Drive, but I was eager to challenge myself.)

The following day -- Tuesday, the morning of my virgin drive -- I left my apartment at exactly 10:20 for my 10:30 a.m. reservation. I was carrying a Uniqlo shopping bag with two pillows I had inherited from my dear, departed friend, Judy, who I had assigned the role of guardian angel.

I entered the elevator, pressed P1, exited the waiting area, and approached the Golf.

My membership card scanned the front window sticker; I opened the front door and placed Judy's pillows on the driver's seat. I tossed my backpack on the passenger's side, and then opened the rear door to lower the back seats.

The two pillows weren't enough to lift me above the steering wheel, so I added my puffy jacket; still not enough. I removed my cellphone and water bottle from my backpack, squished it atop the pile, and pounced on. My heart was beating fast and my mouth was dry. Gulps of water drained the bottle.

The ignition key was latched to the right turn handle, but I was able to insert it. I turned it; interior dashboard lights came on, but no engine noise. I tried again, and again, and again, and then sought out garage personnel.

"Dead battery," said the guy who came to my rescue.

I checked my watch. I had spent 30 minutes in my attempt to start the VW, and would be late for my lunch date if I didn't give up right then. I couldn't believe that all of my preparation, my reconnaissance mission, my two days of pumped-up courage, and my visions of success, proved as useless as the battery.

The company agreed to cancel my three-hour reservation ($41.75 including taxes and fees), and offered a half hour of driving credit. I used a Lyft shared-ride ($15.00) to get me to the restaurant on time.

When I arrived, still carrying the shopping bag and pillows, I proposed using Ruth's car to salvage my practice day. And that's how after lunch, I safely drove her green Honda to her Evanston condo. After hugging her goodbye, I took the Purple to the Red to the Brown line back to Chicago

Next time I seek driving practice, I'll skip the car rental and take the three trains from my place to Ruth's. Perhaps you have an idle car and a destination?

Have pillows; will travel.

PUSHY

"Don't take this the wrong way," my friend said, as she placed a hand on my arm to assure me of her affection. "But, you have a habit of telling everyone how to live their lives. Because <u>you</u> do certain things, you think everyone should follow suit."

I thought for a moment, and then said: "You're right; I'm pushy."

Now that we've gotten that out of the way, listen up: I know what's best for you. In no particular order, here are suggestions -- honed by me -- that can assuage loneliness, lift depression, curb procrastination, improve efficiency, and build self-esteem. (Okay, let's scratch *can* and substitute, *may*. It's possible I'm not actually omnipotent.)

-Write in a journal every morning. I prefer a spiral 6-x-8 notebook and Pilot V Razor Point fine pen. But you can choose your own journal and writing instrument; no electronic devices permitted. A cup of coffee is a lovely companion as you mentally review your previous day and record accomplishments, disappointments, anger, happiness, prideful moments, despair, or anything else that pops into your brain at that early hour.

Important: the journal is for your eyes only, no competition as if you were a member of a writing workshop. This practice is not just for would-be writers; it was extremely therapeutic for me when I was a caregiver for Tommy. My pages were akin to a support group where I could pour out my frustration and fears without getting well-meaning, but ill-fitting, advice from others.

-Enroll in a class or three. Currently, I'm taking lessons in Spanish, piano, and yoga. You may remember that I have attempted these three things in previous years and then abandoned them for one reason or another. No matter, currently, the schedules, locations, and teachers of these disciplines fit into my life. So, I'm back at the chair, bench, and mat. And, along with improving at each, I'm meeting new friends.

I'll throw in another nag here: don't avoid trying something anew because others will remind you that you're previously bailed and re-upped on the very same class. So what; give it a go again.

-Use a timer for tasks. This practice works well for writers who procrastinate about getting anything down on a blank page. But, I also recommend it for those who stall on doing household chores, paying bills, preparing taxes, or any other onerous job.

I use the clock on my iPhone, but a simple, plastic kitchen timer will suffice. Set it for 30 minutes, and then hunker down. When it signals, you are permitted to pop up, and then do something more pleasant.

But, as is often the case with writing, you may find that those 30 minutes have unleashed some buried creativity. If so, you are permitted to silence the buzzer and continue to follow your muse.

-Become a morning person. I realize this will be tricky for those of you who enjoy sleeping late and staying up till midnight. But, if you can massage your body clock to go to bed earlier and rise before sunup, you'll be amazed at the amount of stuff you can accomplish.

I'm not suggesting you incorporate my hours -- 8 pm bedtime and 4 am wake up -- for even I recognize its absurdity. Yes, I need a nap at midday, and ditto to my fading at evening events. I'll trade those hindrances for the calm of being on top of tasks.

-Prepare the night before. This habit works well if you plan to visit a gym in the morning, but find yourself scrapping the goal.

It also succeeds for any other first-thing-of-the-day meeting, class, or appointment. Before going to bed (early, remember?), fill your gym bag with workout clothing, stack your class books and notebook, assemble folders and notes, or gather anything needed to make sure you get out the door on time and arrive prepared.

-Take a walk and talk to yourself. I have a bountiful gym in my high rise, but when weather permits, I do a mile jaunt outdoors. I eschew ear buds and audio, but instead talk to myself. Sure, passersby may think I'm bonkers, but because I live alone, I don't use my voice often enough. Not only does this help vocal cords, but it also forces you to take in your surroundings and perhaps comment, as in: *That's a good-looking grey-haired guy. Wonder if he's got a ring? Maybe I'll smile as I get closer.* (See the possibilities?)

-Express appreciation. If any of my directives feel reasonable, fitting, and potentially fruitful, try my custom: To profess gratitude, send a thank-you note. Electronic can suffice, but handwritten is awesome. (Too pushy?)

HAPPY ANNIVERSARY

"You hit the wrong note."

"Since when do you know piano keys?"

"Don't you remember how much I loved to sing?" Tommy said, as he nudged me over on the piano bench. "You'd play a song from your 'Easy Rogers and Hart,' and I'd croon, like Sinatra."

"Of course, I remember," I said, as I conjured his lean hip next to mine. "You wanted to be a lounge singer, right? It's sad you never got your wish."

"Who's sad," he said. "Do I look sad?"

I lifted my fingers from the piano keys and turned to take him in. It was only his apparition, for he had been dead for more than three years, but I welcomed his occasional appearances with his restored voice.

The image I selected was not the one from his last days in our home with hospice. Instead, I chose his likeness from our wedding day in Las Vegas -- January 13, 1998, 18 years ago.

"Actually, you look happy. Is it because it's our anniversary? Is that why you've dropped in for a visit?"

"Bingo," he said. "Our wedding day was the second happiest of my life."

"And the first?"

"When I met you," he said. "Two years before our marriage."

"It was a whirlwind romance, wasn't it?" I remembered how we had bumped into each other early mornings when he was out for a jog, and I was walking Sasha, my Golden Retriever. When I learned Tommy was about my age, and also divorced, I boldly asked him out.

"One date; that was all it took," he said, turning around on the bench to lean his elbows on the keyboard. "I knew right away I wanted to spend the rest of my life with you."

I was pleased to see him so relaxed. It felt familiar; for Tommy was an easy-going guy. Even when he was challenged by his brain degeneration and aphasia, he was a low-maintenance husband. "So, sweetheart," I said, continuing our chat to keep him near. "I assume you've been monitoring me. What's your view from on high?"

"First the good stuff," he said, as he pulled out a scorecard and pencil before shucking his suit jacket that had the boutonniere still pinned. I smiled when I saw the tiny golf pencil that he often stowed after games. Evidently, Tommy had been keeping score on his wife.

He studied the card and said, "I love that you're still wearing your wedding band. Eighteen years. Quite an accomplishment for a second marriage." Then, he reached over to touch the inexpensive gold ring we purchased at Service Merchandise. His left hand was clear, for I had removed his own ring and saved it with his watch, wallet, and other long-favored possessions.

"So even though you're no longer around," I said, "I should consider us married for the full eighteen?" I didn't think this was accurate, but I liked the sound of it. "Okay, what else is on the plus side of my score?"

"I'm happy to see you at the piano again," he said, "but I don't see much progress." He tousled my hair and smiled, just to be sure I knew he was kidding. "And, I'm relieved you're surrounded by so many friends who care about you. I don't have to worry that you're helpless without me."

"So, I take it you're glad I left L.A. and returned home?"

"Actually, I understood why you moved there," he said. "I saw that my death left a hole in your life and you missed being married. I think you believed your L.A. family could fill that void. But of course, no one could replace me." Then, he rose and danced a bit of a shimmy, as he often did when he wanted to show off.

He placed the scorecard on the piano's ledge so I could read more.

It was lovely to see his familiar handwriting, the same script he used for daily post-it notes to me, and the matching loops and curves in the long, joyful letter he wrote after our wedding.

"Let me play this piece I'm trying to learn," I said. "Remember?" Then, I plunked out the notes to *I'm Glad There Is You.*

Tommy grinned. "Faith and Jill walked me down the aisle to a CD of Johnny Hartman. How could I ever forget?"

As I started to play and sing, *In this world of ordinary people,* I felt a kiss on my cheek and then a draft on the piano bench. "Wait, sweetheart," I said, grabbing thin air. "Happy 18th Anniversary!"

LOSER

As I climbed the translucent steps, I felt as if I were in a 1940's M.G.M. musical. In my mind, I was on a staircase to heaven, with chorus girls in feathery gowns and snazzy guys in tuxedos dancing each tread.

But this was no Hollywood scene. I was at the Apple Store on Chicago's Michigan Avenue, on my way to a 10 a.m. workshop, when I paused to spy on the action below. About two-dozen young people in red logo t-shirts stood quietly while their leader addressed them. As I watched, my mood sagged. *Why can't that be me,* I thought.

My self-pity was not far-fetched because I had indeed been one of them. The year was 2010; I was 72. And after a hiring event at the Old Orchard store, where I had shone in role-playing and interviews, I became a part-time specialist.

"I can't believe it," I said in a three-way call to my daughters. I was about to enter the inner sanctum where my first orientation was to take place, and gushed as if I were an Oscar winner: "I'm surrounded by Macs!"

After I completed the training and joined the team, I scooted the sales floor in my own logo t-shirt and nametag. And despite being the age of my fellow employees' grandmothers, I felt at-home. I joshed with peers as we gathered for our own morning meetings. I excelled at calming older customers who feared technology. And I shared in the excitement of new product launches.

"How can you stand the noise?" I remember my friend Ruth asking on the occasions we'd meet on my lunch hour. I'd look around to view the staff chatting with customers, and realize I had absorbed these sales talks, plus the blares of computers, and heard a symphony rather than a din.

"What noise?" I'd say.

Naturally, I had experiences that weren't favorable. Two have stayed with me. In the first, I was advising a young man on the model of computer that I believed fit his needs. As I pointed out its advantages, he stood with his arms crossed and his face dour. When he wasn't scowling, he was searching the store.

Frustrated, I said, "Is there something wrong? You don't seem pleased with my selection."

"You don't know what you're talking about," he said, "I want someone else."

My reaction was midway between fury and tears. I stifled both and sought out a replacement. As I lingered in the background, I heard my fellow Apple worker recommend the very same Mac. My nemesis clapped him on the back and said, "Perfect." I shook my head and whispered, *Asshole.*

The second blunder was more serious. I had sold headphones to a middle-aged man. For certain small transactions, cash registers were in drawers that sprung out from beneath a display table. "Please stand back," I'd joke to customers, "these can be lethal."

While others laughed, this man reacted differently. "Is it because I'm black?" he said. "If I were white, would you have told me to stand back? Did you want me far from the cash?"

I was mortified. How did my wisecrack go so wrong? I apologized over and over, as wrought as if I had just totaled his car. Eventually, he was mollified and we completed the purchase. We shook hands and he left the store. But I worried he would file a complaint. With my heart beating and hands shaking, I sought out my floor manager. "That's unfortunate," he said, "but I'm glad you gave me a heads-up."

As far as I know, that customer generously forgave me and never tattled. Now I wonder if the incident affected any chance I had of ever being hired again. For recently, I applied for the same part-time specialist job, but instead of Old Orchard, I chose the Michigan Avenue store, walking distance from my apartment.

After a hiring event in September of 2015, I received a, "Sorry, we're going in a different direction," email. Did I lose because I had left my first Apple job after less than six months to be closer to home as Tommy declined? Or, did my former floor manager -- who was now part of the Michigan Ave. crew -- recall the drawer debacle and shut me out? Perhaps, it was just because HR had their pick of hundreds of other candidates who were younger, taller, and smarter than I?

"It's probably for the best," I said to my daughters in another three-way call. "At my age, it'd be tough to stand on my feet for eight hours."

I lied.

HAPPY BIRTHDAY DEAR MOM

"Mom, did you have birthday parties as a child?"
"Oh, it was so long ago, who remembers?"

To make room for her, I scooted over to the corner of my daybed that doubles as a couch. Although my mother died in December of 1981, she annually visits me on her birthday, which is today, January 30.

I loved that she hadn't primped for this pop in. She was wearing a white chenille bathrobe with blue embroidered flowers, and her long black hair with hardly any gray, fell loose down her back. (When Mom was alive, she piled her thin strands atop her head, like movie actresses of the time.) Her face, still absent of wrinkles, lacked her usual rouge, lipstick, and mascara. And the wedge house slippers she wore to add height, were on the floor nearby.

Before reaching over to put an arm around me, she hoisted the stuffed dog that I nightly nestle. "Oy vey," she said, as she tossed it off the bed. "How about finding a guy?"

"Let's not go there." I said. In my mother's dreamy visits, she often worried I would remain single. And although she had a lousy second marriage, to a guy 20 years older than her -- who had her clipping coupons and counting pennies -- she insisted a woman needs a man. "I never want to be a burden to my kids," was how she framed it.

To shift the conversation, I said, "Happy 103rd Birthday, Mom!"

"Shah! That's a horrid thing to say."

"Okay, okay, sorry, no years. I know you never wanted to be an old lady, but I'm just trying to bring us up to date." (Whenever Mom saw a hobbler with a cane or walker, she'd wince. A heart attack just shy of 69 foiled that fate.)

I continued: "So, what I've been pondering, along with my question about birthday parties, is why I was not more curious about your life when you were alive?

"Why did I never ask you about your childhood, your teen years, your relationship with your own mother, romances? Now, all of your siblings are gone, and other than photographs, I have no clue as to who you were before I came along?"

My mother laughed. "You and your daughters put your whole lives out there, so you think anyone who doesn't share is meshugah. Well, some of us are happier being private. Especially in my day; we didn't hang out secrets as if they were damp dresses on a clothesline."

"Nice metaphor," I said, impressed with the imagery. "So, did you want to be a writer, too?"

While I waited for her answer, I nestled closer. I felt her body's warmth and sniffed the familiar scents of her Lux soap and Prell shampoo.

"Writer? That was out of the question in my day," she said. "Back then, as soon as you were old enough -- I was 19 -- you got out of the house and got married. Remember, I had three sisters and four brothers. My mother pushed me towards your father."

"I know the story," I said, glum as I recalled their testy marriage. "I used it in my memoir. When you protested and said you didn't love him, Bubbie said, 'you'll learn to love him.' But, you never did, did you?"

We were both silent for a few minutes. "What can I say?" she said. "We were married for 25 years before he died. He was only 48. You said in your book that I nagged. But if your father had listened to me, had stopped smoking, stopped noshing, paid attention to his diabetes, maybe he would've lived longer?"

"Okay, Mom, this is your birthday. I don't want to bring either of us down. I know you're not going to hang around too long, so before you go, tell me what I can get you as a gift."

"Tell your daughters how much I kvell about them. That would be a gift. Such talent, such good mothers. I'm a very proud grandmother."

"Mom," I said. "Isn't there something you'd like, just for you? I know it'll be make-believe, but I'd like to give you something you've always wanted."

She turned to kiss me on the cheek. Somehow, she had changed her appearance: She now wore face powder, rouge, mascara, and lipstick. Her hair was back in its upsweep.

And instead of the chenille robe, she was dressed in an eye-catching sweater and slim skirt.

"Remember me like this," she said, staining my cheek red. "That's my gift." Then, she swung her legs over the day-bed, slipped into high-heel pumps, and was gone.

POOR BABY

One week ago today, I woke with a sore throat, stuffy nose, and aching head. Because I worried my bug could infect others, at 8:00 a.m., I dressed and slogged to a nearby walk-in clinic.

"Acute upper respiratory infection. It's caused by a virus," the doctor said as he removed stethoscopes from his ears. "Antibiotics won't kill a virus, so I won't be prescribing any. You'll be contagious for the next few days, so it's probably a good idea to stay home and rest."

While I was relieved he had diagnosed nothing more serious than an ordinary cold -- which was likely the same outcome for all of the slumped folks who were stuffing the waiting room by the time I departed at 8:30 -- my illness wasn't serious enough to warrant attention or sympathy. *Poor baby*, I told myself.

(For any evil eyes reading this post, I'm truly grateful my ailment wasn't life threatening, and I am hereby performing *ptu, ptu, ptu* - the simulated spitting that Jewish superstition requires.)

As I walked back to my apartment, where I live alone -- without a husband, without my daughters who live far away, without my mother who is long gone, without friends a door-knock away -- I felt my thirst for sympathy rising with each sneeze. (I know, I know, I could've called you, and you would've rushed over. But, I never want to bother.)

By the time I reached my doorway, I had worked myself into full-blown pathetic. As I unlayered my winter coat, scarf, and gloves, then switched from blue jeans and long-sleeved top to flannel pajamas, I sunk lower into woefulness.

Oh, how I longed for someone to be waiting at bedside to tuck me in, and then pull the covers up to my chin. She, or he, or they, would kiss my un-fevered forehead, ask if I wanted the light on or off, and then tiptoe out. They would close the bedroom door as silently as if an angel food cake were rising in the oven. And later, they would return with a cup of soup or hot tea.

(Because I live in a studio apartment, I'm making up the "bedroom door" bit. In truth, they'd have to retire to a corner. But don't you agree it doesn't evoke the same feeling?)

Since I lacked the power to make any of that nostalgia-driven scenario come true, in this age of social media, I did the next best thing: I turned to Facebook. On my page, I posted this query: "I have an upper respiratory infection; i.e. cold. Advil Cold & Sinus helped, but second dose prevented repose. Up all night. Any suggestions for relief without causing me to be wide-awake again tonight? Thanks!"

Within minutes, the remedies and sympathies came pouring in. At last count, 84 friends had paused their own browsing to offer suggestions. With each comment, I felt as cozy as if they were crowding my bedside.

I imagined them rushing to my apartment with their recommended chicken soup, whisky, zinc, Benadryl, Afrin, Umcka, scotch, humidifier, neti pot, apple cider vinegar, Sudafed, Mucinex, Nyquil, ginger tea, linden tea, and Zicam. I could even envision those who suggested acupuncture dragging along a therapist to perform the procedure. And I could practically hear the water running for the hot bath with Epsom salts another friend believed would cure my congestion.

It was then I realized I had received the *poor baby* I had been seeking. All of these Facebook friends -- admittedly I know only a portion by sight -- were providing my longed-for sympathy and attention. It didn't matter that the succor was virtual, that not a one of them was actually in my apartment; I still felt comforted.

And even though some of the cures were things I'd never try, I enjoyed mentally costuming each of my respondents in a wardrobe that signaled care. Perhaps a nurse's uniform, an herb gardener's green apron, a mad scientist's askew lab coat, a bartender's shirt, or simply a white jacket like the CVS pharmacist who sold me the Advil and Nyquil.

Before complying with the doctor's order to stay home and rest, I purchased a pile of the antidotes on my Facebook list. And, with each spoonful of chicken soup, each thimble of whisky, each sip of ginger tea, my acute respiratory infection slowly dissolved, as if it were the powdered roots in my herbal cures.

So, thanks to the wonders of ancient and modern medicine, virtual and real-life friends, bed rest, and unlimited television, I am just about restored to good health. *Ptu, ptu, ptu.*

ENVY

I had to look up the difference between the definitions of "envy" and "jealousy" because those words were creeping into my head.

I was curious to learn the specific emotion I had been feeling, when I watched a married couple -- a few years older than I -- exchange easy banter.

"Is that what you're wearing?" she had said, her voice interested, but not the least sarcastic. Her look towards her husband carried tenderness, concern, and admiration shaped during a solid marriage of nearly 60 years.

My new friends live in a condominium with a grand piano, captivating views of Grant Park, prized books and artwork, framed photographs of family vacations, and mementos of foreign travel. But none of this abundance was what I envied. *They will grow old together*, I thought. I had no ill will towards them, but I wanted what they had, and that is what is called "envy."

"Jealousy" on the other hand, is when you feel the threat of losing someone, a fear you might be replaced. But since I had already lost Tommy, and it was unlikely he had found another me in his afterlife, I could scratch jealousy as the sensation that had me musing about my friends' coupled life, and my single one.

In the three-and-a-half years since my second husband died, I'd occasionally wake with the notion I wanted a new man in my life. There'd be some void, some bit of the blues, and I'd focus on finding a fella as the salve.

"A companion," I would claim to friends, "not a husband. Just someone for an occasional early dinner, theatre, and perhaps travel. And spooning." I remembered how Tommy and I would fall asleep cradled together like newborn pups.

But whenever I'd toss that notion to friends my age, or to those who witnessed the years of my caregiving of Tommy, they'd return the volley with, "Men your age are not in great shape. Why would you want to take on that burden again?"

"You're right," I'd say, recognizing that my male cohorts aren't as sturdy as their female partners. So, I'd check off, "find a guy," and sign on to multiple interests that would replace that entry.

The hiatus would hold for several months until I'd get the itch again, which led to forays on online dating sites: JDate, Our Time, and Match.com. Bright-eyed, confident, and optimistic, I'd create an honest profile, upload flattering photos, exchange a few witty conversations, meet a handful of men for coffee/lunch/dinner, and eventually flee to "Do not renew" on the membership page.

On the first two sites, I fudged my age by five years, and that brought interested would-be suitors, but none with the glue that survived beyond our first face-to-face audition.

With my latest, Match, the sign-in required my date of birth --1938 -- and instead of fibbing; I fessed up, which became part of my profile.

The men in my selected age range: 72-82, appeared to have slurped from the fountain of youth, for their desired females landed in the 55-65 age group.

So now I've decided -- despite my love for all things techie -- to forgo online dating and stick to a less deliberate method of pairing up. For example, I met my first husband when I was in college and he was dating a friend of mine. He took a shine to me, my friend never spoke to me again, and our marriage lasted 30 years before we divorced.

I met Tommy in 1996-- as the song goes -- on the street where we lived. Rather than an online profile, we easily matched when we learned we were both divorced; and loved dogs, TV, and nights at home. We became a couple after just one date. Before he died in 2012 at the age of 77, his thin brown hair was just starting to show strands of grey; his face just barely creased, and his arms freckled by the hours of golfing rather than age.

If he had lived, Tommy would likely complement my current landscape of lined brow, white hair, and beige dots. And, I'd like to think I'd adore all of his matching emblems. I'd be content seeing us both unvarnished, and blessed with the gift of growing old together -- even with its challenges and complications.

But since that is not to be, perhaps God will place a male in my path. I just hope She doesn't take too long. I worry

Her script might have us meeting "cute," something like a collision of our metal walkers as we tap our way to an early bird dinner.

ONE-OH-SIX

Using both hands, I slide the bathroom scale away from the wall. It is flat, silver-rimmed, angelic, as if no unpleasant news could ever emerge from its opaque surface.

After first resting my palms against the wall to steady myself, I step on the scale. I close my eyes, count to five, and then open to read the digital numbers. *One-Oh-Six,* I say aloud, although no one is in earshot to hear me.

There was a time when that number would have distressed me. It would've sent me rushing to search for a solution that would've lassoed that number and dragged it downward to a desired 100. But now, at age 77, after nearly a lifetime of obsession with my weight, I no longer seek a fix.

One-Oh-Six isn't horrible, I tell myself. I'm only four-foot-nine-inches tall, and those 106 pounds appear to be collecting - as if they were a family reunion of ten generations -- at my waistline. And, in a full-length mirror, my image appears to resemble a water tower. (Instead of H20, my short cylinder is filled with salt, oil, and beef from the Asian dinner the night before. Those were the nasty ingredients that shot my weight up to its current altitude.)

I'm truly grateful that other things have replaced my former weight obsession, including technology. So, if I did a Google search to find a Weight Watchers meeting near my zip code -- just in case -- that'd make sense, wouldn't it? It's the hunt driving me, after all, not the long-erased addiction.

In my morning journal, I record the page number, time, and my weight. I'm a list maker, you see, a writer who appreciates details. With this daily practice, I am able to go back to journals of many years ago and review the events that demanded memorializing. (In November of 2012, 99.)

I drink my black coffee as I write, and after 30 minutes, it's time for breakfast: a quarter cup of orange juice, a half cup of blueberries, one dried prune, four slices of banana, one tablespoon of plain yogurt. This is followed by one-third of a bagel, one teaspoon of original cream cheese, one slice of lox. It feels good being able to eat whatever I want, and to no longer be concerned about the scale.

I'm amused when I think back to the time when my weight mattered to me, unlike this present day. Grade school. Mother. *You don't need that,* she says as she swats my hand from the apple strudel cooling on the stove.

I can't remember, did she then take me to the diet doctor, or was I already in high school when those visits occurred. After weighing in, a nurse would hand out pills for morning, noon, and night, and then schedule the next appointment.

Weight Watchers opened in Chicago in the '70s, and my two daughters would sometimes accompany me to weekly meetings. Is this true, or am I imagining it: did one of them announce to the leader, after I stepped off the scale and was told I had gained instead of lost: *Mommy ate a candy bar.*

My first husband was tall and skinny. I was short and pudgy. (120) Although he and my mother differed on many things, they bonded about my body. Using his nickname for me, he once joked to our daughters as I reached for a slice of cake, *Mother loves her sweets.* We all laughed.

My second husband was short and wiry. A runner and an athlete -- he played softball, ran half marathons, and worked out at the Lakeview YMCA three times a week for 40 years (he was featured in their newsletter). We both became vegetarians; I dropped out after a few months, but Tommy continued the practice until his deathbed. (Now that I think about it, he could've been slightly anorexic in his obsession.) I can't remember him ever mentioning my weight, which I think was around 102 during our marriage and fell to 99 during his hospice.

I know that tomorrow when I step on the scale, the number will likely be One-Oh-Four. And my smart, snickering scale will confirm the two-pound loss.

Although I haven't let the One-Oh-Six bother me, I'm certain I will do what any other rational, self-confident woman will do and simply avoid salty dishes, select fish for a main course, and substitute a half cup of applesauce for the same amount of low calorie frozen yogurt.

It's wonderful to be in my seventh decade, content with my self-image, and not the least bit obsessed with my weight.

MOTHERS

She was sitting in the armchair, her legs stretched out on the footstool.

"Hi, Mom," I said, as I closed the door behind me.

She didn't speak, so I jumped right in. "You're angry, aren't you?"

She sighed. "I guess I should be used to it by now. It seems every chance you get -- first in your memoir, and now on stage, before an audience of 100 people, mostly strangers -- you sneer at my mothering. When are you going to give it a rest?"

"Mom, could we talk about this in my next dream?" I was yawning and tugging off one boot at a time. "I'm so sleepy; it's two hours past my bedtime."

"Poor baby," she said.

My deceased mother visits me often. I hoped I'd be able to get away with the event, which was just a few hours earlier and had focused on my life and my own mothering style.

"Let me see if I can repeat it?" she said. "I've heard it often enough." I sat down on the couch that doubles as a daybed. I leaned back on the cushion, closed my eyes, and listened. Even though my mother was not in the best of moods, I welcomed this chance to hear her voice.

"*I always admired their audacity*," my mother said, repeating the quote that was first published in the Chicago Tribune. I had said that line at the event, referring to my daughters. Mom continued, *"And wish I had it. I grew up more traditional, became a teacher, married a Jewish man at the end of college, and cooked like my mother.*"

I stopped her. "I said 'cooked,' doesn't that imply that I valued your cooking and wanted to emulate it?"

She ignored my interruption, and went on reciting my words. *"When I grew up, my mother decided what I wore, how much I should weigh. I decided to turn it upside down, let my girls choose their clothes, not brush their hair if they didn't want to. They are who I wanted to be. I wanted to be as free as they turned out to be."*

"I noticed you added a new shtick tonight," she said. "*My daughters credit me with raising them to be protagonists in their own stories." (*This had been gifted to me by one of my kids and I used it to show off.)

"Poor baby," she repeated. "You turned out so horrible, didn't you?"

I left my spot and tucked myself in beside her. I put my legs up on the footstool, just like her. "You were a wonderful mother," I said. "It was the times; that's how mothers were back in the '40s. I admitted that in my spiel. I didn't blame you. Did you hear blame in my voice?"

Perhaps I had been a bit harsh. "What part of that hurt you?" I said. "Was it about my weight? You have to admit that you were on me about that."

"I was only thinking about you, about your prospects," she said. She leaned her head against my shoulder. I wished it could linger there throughout the night. "I wanted you to marry well, not like I did. I thought if you were thin, like the models in the newspaper ads, you wouldn't wind up behind a grocery store counter like me. I had bigger dreams for you."

"I didn't know you had dreams for me," I said.

"Not when you were a child," she said. "Remember, when you were 42 and I visited you in your office. You introduced me to your boss. I was squeezing your hand so hard; you had to pull it away."

I was so sleepy. I closed my eyes and conjured the scene. It was 1980, just one year before my mother died at 67. I was working as a communications director for the superintendent of Chicago Public Schools.

"Listen," I said. "I'm so sorry I've hurt you. It's not easy being a mother; I'm sure I've done hurtful things to my own daughters. I just hope they forgive me."

"Does that mean you forgive me?" she said, her voice soft.

"Forgive you? There's nothing to forgive," I said. "You were a wonderful mother; I'm a blabbermouth who fancies herself a writer. Will you forgive me for any words I've written, or said, that have hurt you?"

She smiled, that gorgeous one I so easily remembered. "Of course," she said. "I just wanted an excuse to visit. And by the way, you did great tonight."

With those words, I fell into an even deeper sleep.

COMFORT ZONE

Felix showed me the slot where I was to slide in my two quarters. Then, my seven-year-old grandson skipped away leaving me on my own at the pinball machine. I pulled out the knob near my tummy, watched a tiny silver ball shoot out, and pressed buttons on either side of the cabinet to send flippers flying.

As the glass case lit with each bounce, and numbers racked up to announce my progress, I realized I was having fun. And I had been wrong to protest this evening excursion to a game place I've never coveted. But my main complaint had been I would be taking a predawn plane the next morning, and my comfort zone demanded I be tucked in at that hour.

This experience during a recent five-day trip to Los Angeles followed me home, as if it had been a memento packed in my luggage. I haven't visited a pinball arcade since, but I am still trying to stretch outside my comfort zone.

This change in my rigid behavior got me thinking: when did I first map out this zone, which I had originally thought of as "comfort," but now believe it was more like a corset: tight, restricting movement, impeding breath, and hindering new experiences.

My "sorry, can't do that," usually revolved around time, and my inflexible need to eat dinner at 6 p.m., go to bed at 8, and rise at 4 a.m. This habit was so long-standing that I figured it must have started in my childhood. Surely something that had survived for 77 years -- albeit with minor attempts to break out -- began all those decades ago.

Whenever I talk about growing up in the 1940's, on Division Street in Chicago's Humboldt Park neighborhood, people always respond, "Ah, the good old days." But, I'm quick to correct: "They weren't always so good. Things happened then that weren't sweet and pleasant."

While I hesitate tarnishing anyone's remembrance, in my case, there were episodes that have clung to me as if they were similar to my tattoo, which has faded over the years, but never disappeared. In my memoir, "The Division Street Princess," I describe my parents' contentious marriage; our stateside fear for the safety of uncles fighting overseas, my family's drowning grocery store business, and evil men who preyed on defenseless little girls.

Perhaps it was back then, that I decided it was more comforting to shield myself early in bed, under the covers, protected by my older brother who slept nearby and my parents on the living room's Murphy bed.

Now that I think of it, early bedtimes weren't my only self-imposed confinement. For most of my career, I've been a public relations practitioner, which meant staying behind the scenes and pushing others toward the spotlight.

But that changed in recent years. When my second husband, Tommy, began to decline with brain degeneration, I started writing a personal blog as self-therapy. Slowly, I was starting to tiptoe out, but only on the page.

After self-publishing two memoirs and arranging book readings to push sales, I was forced to move from computer keyboard to lectern, further expanding my comfort zone. I began to say, "yes" to requests to speak before an audience, and two recent events found me center stage.

My latest escape from my inner clock's comfort zone spurred me to enroll in a TV pilot writing workshop that begins at 3:30 p.m. and lasts until 6:30, requiring me to postpone my dinner- and bed-time. While I first hesitated, and balked at the uncomfortable schedule, I've learned that desire eclipses doubt; and dining and retiring later aren't fatal.

And just last week, one of my daughters suggested I attend the performance of her friend who was starring in a one-woman show nearby. The only problem: it began at 8:30 p.m. But, I went. I stayed awake throughout the evening, got to bed at 10:30, and managed to stay asleep until 5:30 a.m. Bolstered by this experience, I've ordered tickets for another one-woman show where the curtain rises at 7:30 p.m.

Based on my history of frequently changing my mind, or leaping before I look, it's possible that one day I'll have journeyed so far from my comfort zone that I become scared, exhausted, or embarrassed, and want to bolt back. If that were to happen, I'll think of my darling grandson and the noisy, darkened arcade. I'll add in a mixed racket of flippers slapping silver balls, people laughing, and remember: I not only survived; I had fun.

COMPOST

I was plopping eggshells and banana peels into the coffee filter -- which already was packed with the morning's grounds -- when I felt a tap on my shoulder. "Compost. Good girl." It was Tommy, who must've sped from his heavenly abode the moment he heard me banging the hardboiled egg on the counter top.

"Hi, sweetheart," I said. "I hate to disappoint you, but no compost here, just an old habit of collecting grounds, peels, and shells for your garden. All this will be tossed in the trash."

"Hope springs eternal," he said. My deceased husband was smiling, likely enjoying this excuse to visit and remind me how clever he was.

"Honey, give up on your wish of turning me into a gardener," I said. "Look around; do you see any bit of greener; a leaf, a flower? That's just not in my DNA."

"Yeah, I remember when we first met. You gave me a tour of your townhouse. I kept my mouth shut when I saw your dieffenbachia, schefflera, palm, and lily. Sad, dusty, neglected. You're lucky you had other redeeming features that kept me from crossing you off my list."

"And when you went straight into the kitchen to find a rag and a pitcher," I said, "I moved you to the top of my list." I remembered how my heart lifted as I witnessed his care-giving. "You dusted every leaf on every plant. You poured life-saving water into each pot. You poked your finger into their soils to make sure they were drinking up."

"Great recall," he said. "I only remember feeling sorry for you; that you had never learned to appreciate greenery."

He had moved to the couch by then, so I hopped aboard, too. "I grew up on Division Street," I said. "Concrete side-walks, no trees, no flowers; that was my landscape during my formative years."

"And that's what I can't figure out," he said, as he put an arm around my shoulder to pull me closer. "Why wouldn't you want to be surrounded by flora now?"

I tried to draw in his scent, to make him more real for me. But my Tommy was a clean freak; showering daily and steering clear of men's cologne. He used an electric shaver, so there wasn't a hint of fragrant cream.

"It isn't a priority," I said. "And when you came into the picture, you brought plants, flowers, and even home-grown food into my life."

"So you remember our vegetable garden?" he said. "Just about this time I'd be searching through the Burbee catalogs. Let's see, we had tomatoes, green peppers, cucumbers, what else?"

I didn't answer for a moment because my memory of those catalogs was tinged with sorrow. Towards the end of his life, when Tommy's brain degeneration had already robbed him of speech and was starting to encroach on his intellect, those pages would accumulate unopened in the wicker basket that held books and magazines. "Too much trouble?" I'd say, when I'd see him toss another onto the pile. He'd nod in agreement.

"Of course I remember our garden," I said. "You always had quite a crop. Your golf buddies and our neighbors would be waiting for their share of your bounty."

He released his arm from my shoulder and leaned back on the cushions, hands behind his head. "What about those peppers!" he said, puffed up as if he were describing a champion offspring. "Spicy as hell, but everyone wanted them."

"I've probably asked you this," he said, "but either I don't remember, or I've chosen to forget your answer. What ever happened to those plants in our house? You didn't just let them fade away again?"

"No, no, I would never do that," I said. "Sara came over with a wagon and took them to her house. She always loved them, and our garden, and you, of course, and she promised to give them a good home."

"Oh yeah," he said, his voice down a pitch, perhaps imaging the wagon, his plants, and their departing. Then he perked up.

"You know, you never really appreciated the whole compost thing. Sure, you contributed eggshells, banana peels, and coffee grounds, but I don't think you understood the beauty of the process."

"So tell me now," I said, happy to find a subject that engaged him and might keep him around a bit longer.

He began a scholarly spiel, which sounded to me like a lullaby. "Well, with compost, we create rich humus for our garden," he said. "This adds nutrients to our plants and helps to retain moisture in the soil." Soon, I was back to sleep.

SHOES

The Nike saleswoman said I could wear my new black/white/dark grey Air Zoom Structure 19 shoes for 30 days. If they were uncomfortable, she promised, I could return them, no matter how beaten up they had gotten. So, with the $130 purchase on my credit card, and my old, brightly colored Sacony Hurricanes in the Nike box, I began my stroll.

Because I'm a goofy sort of person who assigns human emotions to appliances, articles of clothing, furniture, and any other objects, I apologized to my Sacony's.

"I'm sorry," I said, imagining that the gym shoes had been wounded by my new allegiance. Perhaps they were also humiliated by being stowed in the foreign Nike carton. "You're adorable and comfy," I soothed, "but I need a darker pair for dressier occasions."

I can blame my quest for dark gym shoes on my daughter Faith, who worries whenever I wear my black Mephisto sandals with the two-inch wedge heels. Her fear erupted when she and I were walking on the back lot of a Hollywood studio. The sidewalk was uneven, my shoe shimmied a bit, I swayed, and she grabbed me with, "Mom!"

Perhaps my daughter had been influenced by all of the comedies and dramas filmed there, for her horror immediately sped to: "You could fall, break a hip, we'd have to call an ambulance, and you'd spend your vacation in a hospital!"

I had originally chosen the Mephistos because I walk at least a mile a day, and that brand is touted for its comfort. And with the higher heel, I could still look stylish, and taller.

Elevation has long been important to me because I am a wee four-feet, nine-inches. When younger, I made it to four-feet, eleven; but alas, age has elected to chip me away, as if I were a Christmas tree that had to be trimmed to fit through the door.

On fancy occasions, if I were going from apartment to car to venue, I'd swap my Sacony's for dressy high-heeled shoes or sandals. But, as other wearers of these varieties can attest, a good part of those evenings are spent longing for the moment when back at home, we can shuck and walk barefoot.

Recently, on a long walk to visit a friend, I had rejected my Sacony's for a pair of cute Tom's ankle boots with a thick, two-inch heel. They cause no pain; so I figured I could appear taller, and perhaps rise to the height of someone's chest, rather than waist.

Alas, part of my journey included crossing a bridge that had nostalgically retained its original bricks. As I tiptoed across, hands stretched out like an aerialist, I felt myself becoming dizzy. I safely made it to the other side, but vowed not to ever again repeat that path with that footwear.

As you can probably tell, shoes have long been an issue in my life. Actually, shoes + height. I can trace it to my teenage years. During the span, 1952-1956, when I attended Roosevelt High School, in Chicago's Albany Park neighborhood, my chums were shod in white buck.

Because my petite, striving, mother believed I would have a better shot at gaining a boyfriend if I were a few inches taller (slimmer, too, but that's a whole nother essay), she urged a pair of brown shoes with a wedge heel on her obedient daughter.

I'm certain she would've put me out the door in three-inch high heels if she didn't think school authorities would be sending me home with a note, or classmates would jeer.

Oh, I can hear you saying, "Why didn't you protest? Why didn't you tell Min that you preferred trotting the halls exactly as your peers?" If I tell you that not only was I short, but also tender toward my mother, would that satisfy your outrage? I adored her, and would never say or do anything that I believed might hurt her feelings.

Enough psych, back to shoes: After walking the mile back to my apartment in my new black Nike gym shoes ("athletic," if you prefer), I had fallen in love with their look and comfort. The arch is higher than that of the Sacony's, the heel is a tad elevated, and the fashion statement is "damn, they're cute!"

At home, I gently freed the Sacony's from the Nike box, and before placing them back in the closet, offered this: *Sweetheart, please forgive me. We'll meet again when next I walk the park's quarter mile track. Until then, take a break. Gab with the rest of the shoes. Love you!*

Goofy, right?

EXPECTATIONS

Thunderstorms were predicted. The temperature was high in the 90's -- a record for that time of year. Traffic would be horrible, not only was it a Saturday night, but festivals in the city would further choke streets.

Parking would be a nightmare. Many planning to attend would be over the age of 60 and habitually punctual. If they did manage to get to the theatre, they'd surely be lining up long before the start of my 6:30 p.m. show. Would they grumble at the wait? Would arthritic-hampered friends realize an elevator was available that could lift them to the second floor? Why hadn't I noted that in the invitation to my Staged Reading?

Along with those audience concerns, I had promised my cast of 10 there would be no rehearsals. Since they were all actors comfortable performing on stage, and scripts had been in their possession for two weeks, I was confident they'd be at the top of their game. But, what if I was wrong? What if at least one run-through would have perfected the performance of my proposed TV comedy pilot?

This combination of things totally out of my control, plus decisions completely under my direction, combined to find me thrashing nightly in bed, as if I were a canoe battling breakers. Worse, my level of anxiety was threatening to skim the joy from my accomplishment.

Two months earlier, in my customary cheery and naive quest for a new project, I had signed up for an eight-week class at Chicago's iO Theatre. Although primarily known for teaching Improv, iO also offers a script-writing program. I enrolled, eager to execute an idea that had been in my head for several years.

I titled my imagined TV pilot, **Layover**, which told the story of a woman, suddenly widowed and in need of funds, who decides to rent out her spare bedrooms to flight attendants and pilots for their Chicago overnights. While purely fictional, the idea was spurred by a suggestion from a former neighbor who was a United Airlines pilot.

Michael McCarthy, experienced TV writer, taught the workshop, and welcomed me to his group of 20- and 30-year-olds. Because I am a longtime writer, and had previously completed two other pilot drafts, the age difference between my classmates and me wasn't a concern. They were all clever and kind, and I morphed into the dutiful student I've always been, completing homework assignments, refreshing my understanding of the Final Draft script-writing software, and gushing to anyone in earshot about characters and dialogue I thought to be sparkling.

According to McCarthy, our Staged Readings were not to be considered completions, but rather an opportunity to gauge audience reaction and to learn places in the script for polishing or tossing. He encouraged us to invite friends who would populate the 85-seat cabaret, and provide the needed feedback.

This is where I believe my anxiety took root, and then sprouted into an enormous Oak that threatened to burst my brain as if it were an unlucky sidewalk. Heeding McCarthy's suggestion I posted an announcement on my Facebook page, and I sent invitations to 73 friends.

As promises to attend gathered in my e-mail box, I grew tense. What if I had oversold the evening? What if pals were expecting my proposed TV pilot to top earlier books or blogs? What if they assumed my script would flow with brilliant writing, huge laughs, and heartfelt pathos? But what if it was merely mediocre, or worse, what if it stunk? Soon, I became terrified that I would not live up to their expectations.

I considered cancelling, deleting it from my class' calendar. Instead, I summoned courage. There was no turning back; I needed to overcome my fears and produce.

Gratefully, all of my disaster scenarios proved unfounded: There were no thunderstorms. Air conditioning defeated outdoor temperatures. People found nearby parking or took taxicabs or Uber. The elevator was easily marked and accessed.

My stellar cast: Joe Bill, Sophia Mia Canale, Diane Cohen, Tyler Davis, Meghan Flood, Susan Messing, Chuck Otto, Anne Taubeneck, Greg Taubeneck, and Edwin Wald, performed as if we had been rehearsing for months.

Our audience laughed at the right moments, clapped at the pilot's end, and congratulated us for delivering a script and an evening that brought them pleasure. Was my pilot brilliant? Hardly, but hopefully it measured up to my audience's expectations. And for that particular evening, which featured the "Staged Reading of **Layover** -- an original pilot by Elaine Soloway" -- that's all that really mattered.

LONG DISTANCE RUNNER

The number 147 bus travels north along Lake Shore Drive. When riding it, I aim for a window seat on the right side. In this position, if I lift my head a bit, I can see the path favored by runners, speed walkers, and the occasional ambler. Today, lulled by the rhythm of the bus, and the divine Chicago climate, my mind slips from its habit of listing things-to-do, and lands on a figure on the trail. Slowly, with each turn of the wheels of my transit, Tommy emerges.

There is no doubt it is my husband -- deceased, but fully alive in my imagination.

He is wearing a baseball cap to protect his balding head, his feet are in the worn sneakers he prefers, and the radio headphones that covered his ears through his final days in the hospital and hospice, are still in place. I don't want to interrupt his daily exercise, but I assume his appearance means he wants to chat.

"Sweetheart," I say, as I place myself jogging along beside him, "please take off your headphones so we can bring each other up-to-date. (Because this scenario is occurring in my head, I am easily able to speak and trot at the same time.)

My second husband's face is gleaming, partially from sweat and perhaps from joy in seeing me. He doesn't make a move to obey, but continues swinging his arms in a match with his taut legs. "I can hear you, Wifey," he says. "I have special powers now."

"How long have you been running?" I am curious; was he also nearby on Michigan Ave. at the beginning of the bus' route, but there was too much city commotion to spot him? Or, did it take the placid lake and serene setting to bring him into full view?

Gratefully, Tommy has no problem responding. Not only is he not out of breath, as one would expect from a long-distance runner, but the voice that was stilled by aphasia in the last three years of his life, has returned. It is full, alto.

"Oh, I haven't been counting miles," he says. "That's one bonus about the afterlife; no limitations."

"So that means the foot pain that ended your marathons, and made you switch to elliptical machines, is gone?"

"Pain? Sweetheart, we're talking heaven; and, this is <u>your</u> version of heaven. We're in <u>your</u> illusion; you're the writer. You're certainly not going to stage me in poor condition."

"True," I say. "I love remembering you as an athlete. When we first met in 1996, it was early morning, still dark. I was walking Sasha and you were jogging past my townhouse."

"Yeah, I stopped to pet your dog. But I was really thinking, 'who's that cute gal that lives on my block?'"

"Then, Sasha and I -- in the early evening of that same day, when we were sitting on our porch stairs -- we saw you again," I say. "You were on your way to the Y. I was impressed. Quite the athlete."

As the bus continued its route north, I become worried about its eventual turn off the Drive to city streets.

I would likely lose Tommy, because in my daydream, I want him set with the blue sky and matching water, the air free of exhaust fumes, the course empty of stoplights.

"I'm glad you were impressed," he says. "If I remember correctly, you were drinking a beer. I thought, 'hope that cute gal isn't an alcoholic.'"

I laugh at the memory, and at happiness he is still vibrant in my fantasy. "One drink a day," I say, pretending to be offended. "And I never even finish it."

"I'm teasing, sweetheart, only teasing. Just like you, I miss our times together; how easily we got along. I could count on one hand the real arguments we had in our 16 years."

The bus is starting to approach Foster Avenue and I don't want to end my reverie on a scenario that could bring longing, so I back away from nostalgia. "Remember when we jogged together in real life?" I say. "You slowed your pace down to my pathetic 12 minutes a mile."

"Twelve? Wifey, you're really great at painting a rosy picture. It was more like 20." His eyes are twinkling as he says this, and I swear I could feel a gentle poke in my ribs.

And that's where my fantasy starts to fade. The bus is beginning to leave the Drive, so I rush to seal our heart-to-heart. "Drink water!" I say, which must have been aloud because other passengers turn to stare.

FIT

"You crack me up," she said, as she poised mid-fork on a tube of polish sausage she was hoisting to her lips. She was stretched out on our daybed, a wooden tray propped on her lap, and our TV remote was in her left hand.

"I'm glad you find me amusing," I said.

"Oh, come on, sweetheart, you know I'm only teasing." She dabbed her lips with a napkin, and went on. "But you have to admit, we've seen this scenario before."

"Maybe this time, it'll be different," I said, as I continued to arrange equipment I'd need for the following morning. "Ear buds, water bottle, shorts, sports bra, tank top. All set."

"Let's count your gym memberships, shall we?" She ticked off: "There was the East Bank Club, the Lakeview YMCA, Galter Health Center, and one more. Oh, yeah, the Hollywood YMCA when you lived in Los Angeles."

"I'm happy to see your memory is in tact. At our age, shouldn't it be dimming a bit?"

She laughed again, and rose from her prone position to hop on a kitchen stool next to me. I stared at her face, so familiar; for after all, she was I. I was engaged in conversation with upper case and bold ELAINE, the one who has been my nemesis throughout my 77 years.

Instead of praising me for taking charge of my health, this skeptic appears solely to remind me of erstwhile attempts and wimpy abandonments.

"I thought I'd plotz when I saw you with all the pool stuff," she said. "Rubber fins, bathing cap and goggles! Sweetie, how many times have you attempted to swim?"

I don't know why I was trying so hard to win her over; perhaps it was because I craved applause rather than jeers. "The gym and indoor pool are an elevator ride away," I said. I wanted to sound stern, but I fear my voice was more plaintive, so I took the offensive.

"Do you have to eat sausage in front of me?" I said. "You know I'm off red meat." Then I took advantage of her vacated spot on the daybed, climbed aboard, leaned back, and waited for more of her finger wagging.

"Uh, huh, and how long do we think that will last?" With that jibe, she moved to my spot, pushed my extended legs (tauter now, I was sure of it) off our seat, and dropped down next to me. "You're still trying to get rid of this," she continued, poking a finger into my belly. "Blaming this paunch on diminishing height wasn't working for you?"

"Okay, I admit it. When I saw other women my height whose stomachs were as flat as their tushes, I realized I couldn't use my four-feet-nine as an excuse."

She was silent for a moment; perhaps thinking she was coming on too hard. But then, she was on a new tack. "Have you tallied the cost of your fitness toys, togs, and teachers? I thought we were trying to stop spending."

She must've believed I was on the canvas and down for the count, but I had enough stamina (I credit my increased cardio workouts) to punch back. "Okay, the Garmin heart rate monitor was pricey, but it counts my steps, too."

"I recall a few cheap pedometers in your life," she said. By now, she was standing next to the pile of clothing, lifting each one and shaking her head. Then she pulled out a dresser drawer. "Yoga pants? Oh, sweetheart, give me a break."

I jumped up to push her hand away from my wardrobe. "I can also wear these outside the gym and studio," I said. "Workout wear is in."

She smiled, perhaps conceding the point. "Trainer? Swim coach? Nutritionist? How can you justify those expenses?"

"Once a month," I lied. "I want to learn proper technique and healthy eating."

She took this in -- perhaps conceding I had a point -- but then turned her attention to the kitchen. "A vegetable steamer?" She pointed to a recent purchase on the stovetop. "Please don't tell me you're going to try cooking from scratch again."

I was quiet, which may have told her she had gone too far. "Okay," she said, putting an arm around my shoulder. "I'll give you three months. If you're still on the elliptical, in the pool, in the yoga studio, and eating healthily; I'll consider fading away."

"Deal," I said. With that, I gave ELAINE a hug, checked my Garmin, and trotted out the door. Before it slammed, I heard the click of the remote and the sound of a favorite TV show. I hesitated, but didn't turn back. High five!

OVER MY HEAD

Pontoons are used for pleasure boating. They're made out of abrasion resistant PVC and nylon with frames for support and can be equipped with a motor mount, canopy, and a small anchor. Such boats are suitable for seas during calm weather.

One-by-one, my daughters, my grandchildren, and friends who were sharing this pontoon, climbed atop one of it's billowed sides, and leaped into the bay. Only the skipper and I remained.

This bay in Provincetown Harbor is mostly 30 to 90 feet deep, but we had sailed close enough to the shore so that water rose just to neck height of the adults. The children -- all confident swimmers -- gleefully treaded water, or swam underneath to view algae, sea grasses, and fish.

I, the oldest, shortest, and most fearful passenger, was wearing an orange life jacket -- an early bonus from my daughter, Jill, who knew of my unease in deep water.

As I sat, I eyed the calm sea, my carefree loved ones, and with trembling fingers, I untied the jacket. I did not climb the frame, but instead opened the latch of a small door on the pontoon's side.

Everyone in the water suddenly stopped swimming or splashing. They looked up and yelled, "Go, momma, go momma!" So, I did. I jumped overboard, into water over my head. I was able to stroke beneath its surface, move through the algae towards Jill and our other captain, Brandon. As I reached their legs, I felt myself being lifted upwards. "You did it!" they yelled.

Faith joined in, "I'm so proud of you, momma!" I was thrilled, as if I had just won an Olympic competition. "Way to go, grandma!" came from my bobbing grandchildren. And, "congrats, Elaine," from pontoon companions.

With Jill and Brandon at my side, I feebly attempted to tread. But, not wanting to press my luck, I chose instead to return to the boat. I released their arms, and swam a nervous stroke back to the ladder. One foot at a time, I climbed aboard, grabbed a towel, and took a seat as my heartbeat slowly lowered. I had done it; I jumped in and didn't panic.

Like many others who are water averse, it was a near drowning in childhood that turned me into someone afraid of going anywhere near pools, lakes, or boats. I think I was 10; it was at a public swimming pool, its shape starting out shallow on either side, but dipping several feet in the center.

Did I not know that configuration at the time? I can't remember, but the sensation of losing a floor under my wee feet remains clear. Did I flail? Did my friend witness my submersion and alert the lifeguard? Or did that wonderful sun-kissed adolescent spot me among the hundred of kids in the pool that steamy Chicago afternoon and foresee another rescue on his tote board?

I do recall the relief of being lifted out, as floppy as a rag doll, being placed on the pool's cement, coughing out chlorinated water, and hugging the lifeguard as if he were the prince, and me, his just-awakened sleeping beauty.

With that frightening experience, future pool visits were spent solely in the shallow end. And at excursions to North Avenue Beach, I'd venture in the water only up to kneecaps.

For most of my adulthood, my favorite water exercise was finding the perfect spot for a lounge chair or beach blanket. But something changed after I married my second husband. Tommy had been a member of the Lakeview YMCA for 40 years. Because we lived walking distance to that Y, I'd accompany him and work out on the machines or with free weights.

Soon, the scent of the Y's chlorinated pool would tease my nose, but instead of being repulsed, I became intrigued. I signed up for group lessons, learned a feeble crawl stroke, and in the final class, jumped into the deep end and paddled nervously back to the wall.

Attempts at learning how to swim confidently continued at the East Bank Club, Galter Health Center, and now, at the indoor pool of my high-rise apartment building. And that's where I met my latest coaches, first Bill and now

Kathy. Encouraged by her faith in my future as a swimmer, I've been taking her weekly lessons.

Her tips, my Speedo fins and kickboard, and my solo practice sessions have pushed my faith, that this time -- in the 78th year of my life -- I'll claim "swimmer" among my skills.

I have 342 days before our family's possible return to Provincetown, where I pray I'll easily leap off a boat, and serenely swim in water over my head.

TOO MANY COOKS

My mother was the first to appear. "Where's the salt?" she asked, as she steered the bib of an apron over her upswept hairdo.

"No salt," I said. "I'm on a low-sodium diet."

With that, my father leapt to her side. "You think that's bad," he said to his wife, "she's using..." He stopped to pick up the bottle of Extra-Virgin Olive Oil, then continued, "this, this thing, instead of schmaltz."

I knew, when I started cooking my own food, rather than selecting from hot bars at Whole Foods and Mariano's -- as I had done for the first year back in my hometown -- that it wouldn't take long for my deceased parents to pop up in my imagination.

Both died of heart attacks -- Dad at 48 and Mom at 67 -- so naturally, my doctors and I have been vigilant about reversing the family DNA. Admittedly, my guard had frayed at the edges during my year of hot bar browsing. Mashed potatoes, macaroni and cheese, creamed spinach, fried chicken, and Polish sausage had been regular selections.

This salty, starchy smorgasbord slowly added pounds to my 4'9" frame and worse than that, they all took shelter in my stomach. I blamed the balloon at my waistline to diminishing height, and had used rubber bands to stretch between button and buttonhole.

"I think she's doing great." It was Tommy, my second husband who became a vegetarian soon after we wed, and remained thus until he died at 76 of brain degeneration and throat cancer.

My parents -- now surprisingly amiable and agreeable, unlike their 25-year marriage -- moved closer together. "Listen, Tommy," Dad said, "you're a good guy, buy you're a goy. What do you know about Jewish cooking?"

"We love the way you took care of our Elaine," Mom said, "But you're out of your league with Kasha Varnishes." Then, she placed a supportive arm around his shoulder.

"That's where you're wrong, Mom," he said. (My eyes moistened when I heard Tommy call her that. Evidently they've met up in heaven.) Your daughter made that dish for me; it's very vegetarian and healthy, if you make it the right way."

"Look, the recipe calls for 1 tsp. salt," my mother said, as she held up my newly assembled three-ring notebook. "Would that *kleyntshik* amount kill you?"

I paused before answering and enjoyed the image of my dearly departed trio. There was Mom -- not fat, more curvaceous --, Dad, overweight by likely 30 pounds with diabetes adding to his health issues, and Tommy, slender, muscled, and out of this earth before his illnesses had opportunity to vandalize his physique. How I loved, and missed, them all.

"Look, sweethearts, I know you have my best interests at heart, but I believe I'm on the right track." I removed my apron, placed my hands on my hips, and did a runway walk. As I sashayed, my palms moved to my stomach. "Gone," I said. "My two months of low salt and no red meat, plus daily exercising have drained seven pounds of fat -- nay, schmaltz -- from my body. I feel terrific!"

My parents took a seat on my daybed. "No red meat?" Dad asked.

"Pastrami, corned beef, all deli, all gone." Mom said. She shook her head, looking as disappointed as if I had switched allegiance from Hadassah to Daughters of the American Revolution.

I perched on a stool next to my island counter. "You'll all just have to assume I know what I'm doing."

"You're going to waste away to nothing," Mom said, her blues eyes downcast.

"Do I look malnourished?"

"You could be a bit more zaftig," Dad said.

"Mom, Dad, she looks great," Tommy said. "And, she visits her doctors regularly, so they'd catch anything that doesn't look kosher."

Both of my parents sat erect from their relaxed positions on the daybed. "Kosher, he said! Our son-in-law said, 'kosher.'"

Now the conversation between the three of them was warming up. "Your daughter introduced me to plenty of Jewish foods," Tommy said. "Of course, I asked her to convert your chopped liver recipe to vegetarian."

My father took out a handkerchief and wiped his brow. My mother closed her eyes. Was she crying or laughing?

"Extra virgin olive oil, onion, toasted walnuts, hard boiled eggs, canned peas, salt and pepper to taste," Tommy said.

With that, both of the apparitions of my parents vanished. I could hear faint laughter accompany their disappearance.

"Hold up, time for me to go, too," Tommy said, waving an arm to empty air. Then, he patted my tush, and whispered, "zaftig enough for me."

SHOWBIZ

The nurse and I are attempting to raise the head of my bed so I can watch the traffic in the aisles of the emergency room. She's unpracticed, so we wave over the doctor in the next bay and he figures out how to lift me for a better view.

We are not really nurse, patient, and doctor, but instead, "Extras," or they say in showbiz, "Background." The three of us, along with another 50 or so of our ilk: curious folks who signed on for a kick, partially employed people who do it for extra cash, and TV star wannabes who dream they will be plucked from our troupe for a speaking role.

No matter our motive, all are friendly; a majority know each other from background work on various other TV programs now being filmed in Chicago. We had all answered the call issued by Tall Sticks Casting for scenes in the popular Dick Wolf show, Chicago PD. But because this episode has a storyline that involves a wounded officer, it is a crossover with Chicago Med, hence the nurse, the doctor, and me, the patient in the bed.

I had submitted my name, photo, age, dimensions, and other data for a day that needed people of all ages (hand raised). I thought I'd have a shot because there'd unlikely be other 78-year-olds willing to be at the studio (Cinespace) by 6 a.m., schlep outfits to befit a patient, or waiting room sadsack, and be available for 12 hours or more.

When I got the email telling me I had been selected, I immediately forwarded it to my daughters, who are successful TV writers and directors. "How exciting!" they wrote back, with a flurry of exclamation points matching my own.

I knew my kids would be happy about my little showbiz fling because they were the ones who had set my brain to fame. Jill, who created the Amazon Prime streaming video, Transparent, and Faith, a member of her sister's writing team, invited me to appear in a cameo -- with lines! -- in an episode of the show's third season, which both daughters wrote.

There are photos of me outside a trailer with a poster of my name on its door. That's me in another trailer with makeup and hair artists prettying me up for the harsh lights of the set. Then, there was the actual scene where I played a member of a synagogue board with several of the show's stars.

Although I had memorized my lines, Jill the director, suggested we throw in some improvisation. So, the final words that appear in the scene are a mix of my daughters' and mine. I downloaded the new season as soon it was available, eagerly watched the first two episodes, and then zeroed in on the third with a scientist's focus: *Do I look okay? Are my eyes open, or did my eye tick distract? Is my dialogue intelligible?*

While I was satisfied I wasn't an embarrassment to my daughters, my first reaction was like a jealous diva: *That's it? Why couldn't the camera linger a bit more on that interesting grey-haired woman?* I wanted to hear more of her opinion; surely the audience felt the same.

Oy, I had been bitten by the showbiz bug, and that's how I wound up with a hospital gown tied over my white t-shirt and gym shorts, lying propped up on a bed in the emergency room of the fictional Gaffney Chicago Medical Center.

While lying there waiting for the director to shout "Action!" I pondered: *If I were a real patient in an E.R., shouldn't I be alert and surprised at the tumult when the police and medical teams barrel through the aisles? But, if I sit up with a quizzical look on my face, would the director choose to scrap my image?* I elected to remain in my upraised position.

The new season for Chicago PD just started, so my appearance (or lack of) won't show up for a couple of weeks. Unlike my cameo in Transparent, where ahead of time I continually gushed to friends on social media to keep an eye out for my close-up, for this latest role as a background patient, I'm keeping mum. It's likely in that rushed scene; the camera won't absorb the elderly woman propped up in bed, whose face hauntingly evokes fright and curiosity.

Showbiz can be such a bitch.

OBSESSED

Dear blog fans: I apologize for not publishing a new post this week, but I'm unable to move from my anti-Trump obsession to consider anything else. You see, I traditionally elect an essay theme with this question: "What has been going on in my life that is relatable and universal?"

At times, I thought I'd write about my swimming progress, or my functional strength training, or about my return to Saturday morning Torah study, or the recurrence of sciatica in my right leg.

But, the minute I'd sit down at my MacBook Air, with the screen opened to Word, my anti-Trump mania -- as if it were a careening truck of dynamite -- slammed into those ideas and knocked them flat.

My obsession has caused me to assess old and new friendships. With the former, whom I know are anti-Hillary Clinton, I have taken a break from our long-time relationship and hopefully, will resume post election. Because I have not heard from this friend, I assume she has decided on the same path.

For potential new acquaintances, wait; let me give you a *for instance*: I was seeking a seat at High Holiday services when I spotted a woman about my age sitting alone. "Do you mind if I sit next to you?" I asked, assuming she'd be pleased with the company.

She was. "Of course, sit down," she said. We introduced ourselves, and for a moment she was in a good light. When a friend approached and congratulated me on my daughter Jill's recent Emmy, my potential pal lit up. "Tell me all about it," she said. Of course, I did.

But alas, I made the mistake -- wouldn't you have assumed the same, sitting in a Reform synagogue that all parishioners shared your beliefs -- of bringing up the subject of the presidential election. She began okay, listing Trump's negatives, but then said the fatal words: "I can't vote for Hillary; she's awful, too."

Like the Torah scroll that would soon be opened and then, closed; I rolled shut our conversation, and turned to my left where I found an old friend with the exact same views as mine. The next week, when I saw the now, polluted-parishioner sitting solo, I moved to a different row.

The coming election has altered my morning routine. Instead of checking my Gmail account first thing in the morning, I race to websites for the New York Times (long-time print and online subscriber) and the Washington Post (a recent online edition customer).

If I spot an article that fits my viewpoint and deserves sharing with my social media followers, I immediately select a tantalizing paragraph, copy and paste, and publish. Only then, can I enjoy breakfast.

And when I encounter a link that a Clinton supporter has posted, I speedily share. I've been astounded, but not surprised, following the Trump "locker room" video, at the number of women who are raising hands to divulge their experiences of sexual harassment and abuse. Count me as one who has endured, and wrote about it in my memoir, "The Division Street Princess." (The multitudes are not a surprise, for whenever I discuss my memoir in college classrooms, the majority of young women -- decades after my experiences -- sadly describe their own.)

My iTunes Library is being tapped more now. Previously, when unloading the dishwasher, preparing salads, or doing other mindless tasks, I would routinely have MSNBC chatting on my Samsung flat-screen. But now, whenever anchors or commentators shift from anti-Trump to anti-Hillary, I reach for the remote and send them sailing.

I'm calmer, with the crooning of Carmen McRae, Ella Fitzgerald, Johnny Hartmann, Billie Holiday, Barbara Cook, Dianne Reeves, Ernestine Anderson, Etta Jones, Lucinda Williams, Mandy Patinkin, Nina Simone, and Shirley Horn. (OMG, I hope none of those who are alive are Trump supporters. If so, they'll have to be bypassed until after the election. It would be painful to eliminate them completely.)

So, dear blog fans, I hope you forgive me for not writing a new post this week. Soon enough, I'll bring you up-to-speed on my swimming progress, or my functional strength training, or about my return to Saturday morning Torah study, or the reoccurrence of sciatica in my right leg. But for now, not one of those topics has a chance of overtaking my obsession. Thanks for understanding.

DENSE

He was stretched out on a lounge chair, snoring, with a lit cigarette dangling over a nearby potted plant. "Daddy," I said, as I entered the indoor pool, "you're not supposed to be smoking here."

My raised voice startled my dad. He woke, pushed the stub into the plant's soil, then smiled and said, "Good morning, Princess."

I wasn't surprised to see my deceased father because on practice days I call out to him: "Please clear the lanes of swimmers." I say this before leaving my apartment; my eyes upwards. My father often boasted he swam at the Division Street Y with Johnny Weissmuller -- later known as Tarzan -- so; I've picked Dad to hear my plea.

"What persuaded you to appear this morning?" I said to the apparition, as I unpacked my mesh bag. My heart bobbing with happiness.

He laughed -- oh how I remember that smile, and those teeth, which nightly floated in a glass on our bathroom sink. "*Gavalt*," he said, as I dropped to the pool tile: fins, kickboard, bathing cap, goggles, and water bottle. "What's all that mishegas?"

"I use them for my drills," I said. "My teacher Kathy thinks this stuff aids my practice. Have you been here during my lessons? I've never felt your presence."

"No, Princess, I leave you to her when she's with you. But, I do hang around when you're alone, just to keep you safe. I'm in the whirlpool."

I turned to the tub and imagined Daddy basking in the cloud of bubbling steam. He must've been hidden by the vapors. "So, why do you appear today?"

"I just wanted to let you know how proud I am, that you're continuing to learn to swim."

I wanted to go in for a hug. But I knew better than to approach an imaginary Dad. What if I crossed some metaphysical boundary that would make him disappear? No, I thought it best to continue our conversation with him in the chair, and me in the water.

"Why are your legs dangling?" he shouted. I always start my time in the pool with some easy floating. This is what he must have been referring to.

I stood up in the water -- it's only 3'6", so not a feat -- lifted my cap from my ears, and pushed my goggles to the top of my head. "What did you say, Daddy? I couldn't hear you."

By now, Dad had risen from his lounge chair, re-buckled his belt, which in my memory was always unloosened when at home he settled in with Camels and paperback. "Your legs should be straight out," he said, demonstrating with flat hands.

"My body is too dense," I said, boasting as I flexed calf muscles. "It's okay to float in this position; it's still considered floating."

"Dense," Dad said, laughing, "that's a new one on me." He raised both arms, shot up biceps and said, "These never stopped me from floating."

I looked at his belly, still full and round, but decided not to point out this flotation aid.

"Speaking of dense," I said, "I feel dense, dumb, about you. Who were you in your youth? Why didn't I ask you about your teen years, the years before Mom, before Ronnie, and me? And you die when you're just 48? I never got a chance to fill in the blanks."

"What's to tell?" he said, as he removed shoes and socks, and rolled up his pants. As he sat on the pool's ledge, dangling his feet in the water, he continued: "I had buddies. We played baseball -- I was pretty good. You know I didn't even go to high school. I worked. I had to help support the family; we were eight kids."

"But what were your dreams, your ambitions? You ran the grocery store, butchered meat. Was that what you wanted out of life?"

He swirled his legs, making waves in the water. "I wanted to be a writer," he said. "Remember all the books I read? Mickey Spillane?"

"I'm a writer!" I said. "Ronnie's a writer! My girls write! So, that's where we get it from."

He smiled and splashed his feet, then became serious. "But, I had to make a living. The store did that for a while.

I was happy, all of us together. Mom and me at the counter. You at your little sundries department, and Ronnie making deliveries. It was my new dream."

To comfort him, I paddled over and reached to touch his leg. As I feared, he disappeared. I replaced my cap, and the goggles covering my misty eyes. Then stretched out in the water, floating, with dense legs dangling.

VOICES

Both of my spouses were confident and talented singers. My first has a beautiful tenor voice and during our marriage, she took weekly lessons; opera was her repertoire of choice. (When we were together, she acted as a man. Now, she is living her true self as a transgender woman.)

My second husband Tommy also had a lovely -- a more cabaret voice -- and although he died in 2012, I like to think of him still singing around a celestial piano.

My spouses' voices came to mind because I'm currently taking lessons. Perhaps my envy of their ease with singing sparked this new quest. I have no desire to perform, but since I can, sort of, play Broadway ballads -- admittedly in my own tempo -- I want to sing along as I plunk.

I told my new voice teacher that I signed up because I couldn't sing. After a few basic exercises, she said, "Who told you that you couldn't sing?" I smiled, as happy as if she had announced I won the lead in a popular musical.

"I can sing well enough when elbow-to-elbow with someone who has a strong voice," I told her.

"But in a previous class, when I had to sing solo, my voice ricocheted." I was trying to be funny, but whenever I think about that time, I still feel embarrassed and disappointed.

"Singing is a skill that can be learned," she said. "All you need is pitch, practice, and confidence."

Because I have progressed -- albeit to a satisfyingly mediocre level -- in lifelong pursuits like piano, swimming, and Spanish, I believe the same path might apply; hence my enrollment in private study at Old Town School of Folk Music.

If I learn some of the skills, and if I practice, perhaps I can be a so-so singer. That would make me happy.

Now, I'd like to tell you more about my spouses and their voices. My first's foray into singing on stage came during a brief time our family lived in a suburb of Chicago. We had joined a community theater group, and she played leading roles in several Gilbert and Sullivan musicals. I stayed behind the scenes.

When my family left the suburbs and moved to South Commons, a community on Chicago's near south side, I recalled my spouse's enjoyment of performing, and I persuaded the ecumenical minister in charge of programming, to launch a musical theater company.

The South Commons Musical Theater mounted several Gilbert and Sullivan operettas, and a few Rogers and Hammerstein classics. In my favorite, "Carousel," my spouse took the role of Mr. Snow, and our daughters (about eight and nine years old) joined her on stage as Snow's children.

Alas, neither Gilbert, Sullivan, Rogers, or Hammerstein could save our marriage; we divorced after 30 years.

But I married again, in 1998 to Tommy, who loved to sing but never aimed for the stage. His favorite spot was standing next to our piano crooning, "Blue Room," while I plodded along key by key. Once, I asked him what career path he wished he had taken. "Lounge singer," he had said, his face lit as if a spotlight was already focused on him.

Ironically, this sweetheart who loved to use his voice, in 2009 developed a brain degeneration that eventually robbed him of all speech; and cruelly, song. Oh, he did have several sessions with a therapist to see if she could tug words from brain to mouth, but any progress was crushed by a more powerful foe.

Tommy died four years ago and his framed photo sits atop my upright. I begin each practice session with a wink to him and then a leap into syllable sheets that has me stretching through do, re, mi, and more. Once warmed up, I turn the pages of my three-ring binder to songs previously practiced with my piano teacher.

I play and sing my repertoire, which includes: "Bewitched," "When Sunny Gets Blue," "It Never Entered My Mind" (Tommy's and my favorite), "I'm Glad There is You" (I marched down the aisle to this), "But Not For Me," and "Blame It On My Youth." I can hear you humming along, dear reader. It's lovely to croon, isn't it?

Now that I'm taking voice lessons, I try to sing loud and confident, not worrying if the notes are a bit askew. Neighbors on my high-rise floor, on their way to the trash chute or elevator, can likely hear me. Some may shake their heads at my amateurish belting, but no matter. My voice teacher told me I can sing.

RING FINGER

I couldn't decide between a 14" chain I already owned, and the 18" gold-over-sterling silver that I eyed online. Because the longer one was inexpensive, I opted to order it, figuring that if I disliked it, I could use it for some other dangle.

In the three days that my ring finger has been absent of my wedding band, I have used the 14" one to hold it. Although the chain feels a bit snug, a bit too close to the neck, I still wear it 'round-the-clock, just as I have done ever since Tommy and I married in 1998, and beyond his death in 2012. In all these years, the ring had never left my finger, until now.

During those 18 years, the band (purchased from Service Merchandise for $25) has narrowed the skin of my finger so that, minus it, the digit appears misshapen. Perhaps in time, without its wrap, the pinkie's partner will fill out and look like its four brethren.

There are actually two reasons I removed the ring and placed it on a chain. You may prefer the first because it is true; or you'll opt for the second, which embarrassingly, is also true.

The initial motive was prompted by two recent occurrences: swimming four days a week; and through healthy eating, losing 10 pounds in five months. Lately, my wedding band had become loose on my finger, as if it had been coated with WD-40. I worried that on one of my sloppy strokes, the ring would slither off, and I'd have to scuba to the pool floor to find it.

The thought of not wearing my wedding band was unbearable; I could not dishonor a beloved husband and our easy-going marriage. So, I searched a drawer where I stow my jewelry and discovered the 14" chain that held a charm of a lion. Because my birthday is in August, I think the neckpiece and the Leo zodiac must've been a gift from my first spouse. It had been stored -- not because of any animosity towards her -- its just I seldom wear jewelry, save for earrings, and of course, the wedding band we're discussing.

When I found that 14" chain, and slipped off the tiny lion head, I realized the irony: I was deleting a keepsake from one partner and replacing it with one from another.

I'm assuming you're content with my explanation of a wobbly ring, swimming practice, and the possibility of loss. Perhaps you're even teary-eyed as you witness me fondling the band dangling from my chain. But because I've always tried to be honest with you, I'll confess to reason number two for the ring's removal: I'm opening myself to dating and reckon a gold ring on my left hand signals married status, and therefore unavailable.

I've landed on that theory because on my daily walks or at events, I eye grey-haired men who appear to be my age. After verifying neither a spouse, walker, or cane accompanies him, I focus on the left hand: banded or blank?

Now, he could be a widower with loyal feelings toward his deceased spouse, and still wear the wedding band -- just as I had done till my recent removal. But, I'm guessing that men, without the social support of a wife, return to the hunt sooner than women, hence a quicker removal of the telltale band.

Admittedly, it could be reasons other than my ring that have kept prospects at bay. There's my authentic gray hair, wrinkles resembling crossword puzzles, arm flesh flappy as a flag, and other realities of an unvarnished aging life. And because healthy, single, older men are a desired demographic, they have their choice of women 10 years younger (20?) than themselves, sans all of the eyesores I've just described.

But, despite my confessed challenges, and my contentment with my single life, something is kindling a desire to be coupled. Not married -- two musically accompanied walks down the aisle have been sufficient -- but a companion, pal, dinner date, or cuddler would be nice.

When the 18" chain arrived, with difficulty, I unclasped the shorter version, slipped off the ring, dropped it through its new home, and with more difficulty (hence the need for a companion to assist clasping and zippering) fastened it. This length works better; it doesn't feel as restricting as the first.

And, because I often feel the ring still on my finger, somewhat like the sensation of a phantom limb, when I glance at my left hand, I startle: *Where has it gone?* Then I remember: It has been relocated to a new home -- closer to my heart.

RING FINGER, PART TWO

"No, no, don't open that box."

"But your ring could be in there," I said. "I remember I looped it around your watchband and stored it with your stuff."

"I'm warning you," he said. "It's not there."

I ignored my deceased husband's advice because for one, he was not actually present: he was a figment of my imagination that occasionally pops up. And, secondly, I was certain I had packed the ring with his ashes.

I was on a search for Tommy's wedding band because after writing an essay about how I had removed it from my ring finger to prevent its loss while swimming, I lost it.

"You shouldn't have used that magnetic clasp," Tommy said. "It was bound to open and send your ring sliding off."

"You weren't around to hook the chain," I said, as I dragged over a stepstool to reach a closet shelf. "I added the magnetic clasp so I could do it myself."

As I placed the USPS box on the island counter, Tommy stretched out on the Ikea daybed that doubles as a couch. He put his arms behind his head and hummed, "When The Saints Go Marching In."

"Very funny," I said, pulling apart the shipping tape that had reattached itself after the box was first opened.

"You know what you're going to find," he said, taking a break from his song. "Did you think it would miraculously get cleaned up?

In the middle of the shipping carton stood a dark brown box decorated with autumn leaves; it held my second husband's ashes. Well, it was supposed to hold onto them on its ride from Los Angeles to Chicago. But, in the bounces from truck to plane, from one delivery guy to another, the container unfastened and grey ash covered everything.

When I first saw this more than a year ago, I closed the carton unfazed. In my heart, I knew the ashes were merely an earthly reminder of Tommy, and that the majority of his ashes were spread in beloved places: the park near our home on Dakin St., outside the Lakeview YMCA he frequented for 40 years, and near the spot in Jackson Park where he got a hole-in-one.

The few ounces that were left were now coating his wallet, an old framed photo of his softball team; but not the watch with his ring looped through.

When I lost my ring, I searched everywhere: pool, elevator, hallway, apartment; but it was nowhere to be found.

I have an uneasy suspicion that in the bathroom, after I had peeled off my bathing suit, and heard a mysterious clink, it was the ring travelling from its opened chain, down my chlorine-coated body to our city's sewer system.

Rather then lamenting my loss, and its likely solo swim, I opted to find Tommy's band and use that on the 18-inch chain. This time, I would use its original clasp, forgoing the magnetic one that led to my ring's dismal departure.

"It's in the top drawer," Tommy said, pausing his song and adding a told-you-so grin.

He was right; in the back of the drawer, in a plastic baggy, was the watch and ring.

"Apologies," I said, as I lifted his wedding band and slipped it through the chain. Miraculously, I now could reach behind my head, find the tiny circles with my pinched fingers, and securely seal the chain.

"Much better," Tommy said. "You should've been wearing mine instead of yours in the first place."

"You're right," I said. "But I'm glad I did it the other way around, otherwise it would be your wedding ring that had disappeared."

Tommy started to laugh. "You know I read in your blog that another reason for taking off your ring was to lure a guy to your life. You little flirt," he said.

I quickly stopped what I was doing, rushed to the daybed, and jumped on his lap. "Hubber," I said, "that was all for comic effect. You know I'd never try to find your replacement. Impossible."

Tommy became serious. "It has been four years," he said, "and I'm not surprised you'd get lonely. But, I wouldn't be honest if I didn't admit it stung a bit; I hoped I'd be your last love."

"No worries," I said. "I've already dropped that idea. When I thought further, I realized it would be more nuisance than I was willing to accept."

With that, Tommy touched the 18" gold-over-sterling silver chain that I now wore around my neck. He patted his own wedding band. "Looks good," he said. Then, he was gone.

CAN LIVE WITHOUT

It was five a.m., and out of habit, I strolled to my front door to seek the sliver of shadow alerting me that the New York Times was waiting on the other side. But all I could see in the gap between door and floor was light coming from the hallway.

It was then I remembered I had cancelled the paper's home delivery and switched to online.

This change wasn't based on a desire to be environmentally conscious and reduce the number of trees required for my daily papers. Instead, it was one of many cut backs I was forcing on myself to save money.

For the past three years, I have been living in pricy apartments and spending madcap, as if I were an heiress with unlimited funds instead of a jobless, 78-year-old widow with occasional gigs and a dwindling retirement account.

But lest you shed tears at that dour description, remember I am blessed with two daughters who have vowed to help or house me when my balance sheet flattens. And, I'm aware that many are in true poverty, and I am a person of privilege. Thus, I'm not seeking sympathy.

Actually, what I need from you is encouragement. Something along the lines of: *You've done it before, Elaine; you can do it again. You're a sharp cookie; you'll make a frugal plan and stick to it.*

Thanks for reminding me that I had indeed donned this fiscal corset in another point in my life, and that experience turned out well. Interestingly, the previous belt-tightening, and the current one, have something in common: both were spurred by the tug of Home.

My first penny-pinching plan took place 22 years ago. After a divorce in my first marriage -- although left with a fair sum -- through careless spending, I became $35,000 in debt. This predicament forced me to sell my home. With the sale, I paid off the tab and rented a trendy loft apartment in River West. Unfortunately, this move did nothing to alter my habit. Instead of credit cards, I now used house-sale profits to finance my life style.

A few years into my lease, I decided I wanted to be a homeowner again. But at the rate I was tapping my savings, I wouldn't have enough for a down payment. I found a row house under construction in Lakeview and had six months to prove I could survive on my public relations income.

I read books on living as a tightwad, perused business and money sections in the newspapers, and dropped all spending I categorized as "Can Live Without." By the time my coveted house was ready for move-in, I was free of debt and had my signature on a mortgage.

My newest quest to curb spending was sparked by this realization: If I continue to draw from my retirement account at the same rate I have been doing, I will run out of money in about five years.

My first thought was the simplest: Move. I live in an expensive studio apartment in downtown Chicago. Surely I could find a place somewhere in the city that would be hip, and half my rental fee. But the more I pondered that thought, my mood shifted from grit to grim. I cried at the thought of leaving my adorable cocoon and lovely high-rise with concierge, a maintenance staff, and indoor swimming pool and gym. I'd miss my proximity to doctors and hospital and my Michigan Ave. jaunts. So, that's when "Can Live Without" plan #2 went into force.

Thus far, along with switching from the New York Times' print to online -- which is saving me $50 per month -- I cancelled a class I had enrolled in at Old Town School of Folk Music ($186) and a woman's retreat sponsored by my synagogue ($350).

I cut monthly expenses by dropping in-home massage ($80), personal training ($120), switching hair cuts from salon to barber shop ($80 reduced to $33), eliminating Adobe Pro DC ($14.99), suspending Dropbox's Pro ($9.99), patronizing Trader Joe's more often than Whole Foods ($100), declining most lunch invitations ($200), reducing charity contributions ($81 to $18), and avoiding mindless clothes shopping ($115).

You'll have to do the math because I'm too lazy, but I think you'll agree that I've already sliced a significant sum from my outlay. So, if I can steadily spend $500 less each month that means my retirement account plus Social Security will buy me more time and I can stay put. Maybe I can even add years to the day when my dear daughters open their door and find Momma -- not the Times -- at their doorstep.

Made in the USA
Middletown, DE
24 May 2024

54796135R00159